COMPACT *Research*

Alzheimer's Disease

by Peggy J. Parks

Diseases and Disorders

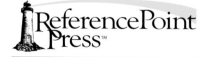

ReferencePoint Press™

San Diego, CA

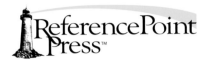
ReferencePoint
Press™

Picture credits:
Maury Aaseng: 33–36, 49–51, 65–68, 82–85
AP Images: 11
Science Photo Library: 15

Parks, Peggy J., 1951–
    Alzheimer's disease / by Peggy J. Parks.
        p. cm. —(Compact research)
    Includes bibliographical references and index.
    ISBN-13: 978-1-60152-061-6 (hardback)
    ISBN-10: 1-60152-061-1 (hardback)
    1. Alzheimer's disease. I. Title.
    RC523.3.P37 2009
    616.8′31—dc22
                                                    2008027935

Contents

Foreword

As modern civilization continues to evolve, its ability to create, store, distribute, and access information expands exponentially. The explosion of information from all media continues to increase at a phenomenal rate. By 2020 some experts predict the worldwide information base will double every 73 days. While access to diverse sources of information and perspectives is paramount to any democratic society, information alone cannot help people gain knowledge and understanding. Information must be organized and presented clearly and succinctly in order to be understood. The challenge in the digital age becomes not the creation of information, but how best to sort, organize, enhance, and present information.

ReferencePoint Press developed the *Compact Research* series with this challenge of the information age in mind. More than any other subject area today, researching current issues can yield vast, diverse, and unqualified information that can be intimidating and overwhelming for even the most advanced and motivated researcher. The *Compact Research* series offers a compact, relevant, intelligent, and conveniently organized collection of information covering a variety of current topics ranging from illegal immigration and methamphetamine to diseases such as anorexia and meningitis.

The series focuses on three types of information: objective single-author narratives, opinion-based primary source quotations, and facts and statistics. The clearly written objective narratives provide context and reliable background information. Primary source quotes are carefully selected and cited, exposing the reader to differing points of view. And facts and statistics sections aid the reader in evaluating perspectives. Presenting these key types of information creates a richer, more balanced learning experience.

For better understanding and convenience, the series enhances information by organizing it into narrower topics and adding design features that make it easy for a reader to identify desired content. For example, in *Compact Research: Illegal Immigration*, a chapter covering the economic impact of illegal immigration has an objective narrative explaining the various ways the economy is impacted, a balanced section of numerous primary source quotes on the topic, followed by facts and full-color illustrations to encourage evaluation of contrasting perspectives.

The ancient Roman philosopher Lucius Annaeus Seneca wrote, "It is quality rather than quantity that matters." More than just a collection of content, the *Compact Research* series is simply committed to creating, finding, organizing, and presenting the most relevant and appropriate amount of information on a current topic in a user-friendly style that invites, intrigues, and fosters understanding.

Alzheimer's Disease at a Glance

What It Is

Alzheimer's is a progressive, irreversible, and fatal disease of the brain. It is part of a family of diseases known as dementia.

Prevalence

An estimated 26 million people throughout the world suffer from Alzheimer's, and 5.2 million live in the United States.

Cause

Scientists do not know exactly what causes Alzheimer's disease, although they suspect that numerous factors are involved, including genetics and environment.

The Hallmark of Alzheimer's Disease

The brains of people with Alzheimer's become clogged up with abnormal structures known as beta-amyloid plaques and neurofibrillary tangles. Whether they are caused by the disease or are by-products of it is not known.

Symptoms

Alzheimer's causes memory loss, confusion, disorientation, and radical personality changes that can lead to inappropriate or even abusive behavior. As the brain continues to deteriorate, symptoms grow more severe.

Cause of Death

Alzheimer's is always fatal, but people rarely die from the disease itself. Brain atrophy severely weakens the body, which makes patients susceptible to pneumonia and infections.

Treatment

No proven treatment can stop the progression of Alzheimer's disease, but some drugs and lifestyle changes have been shown to delay symptoms and provide comfort.

A Looming Health Crisis

If a cure is not found, the Alzheimer's Association predicts that the number of people with the disease could reach 7.7 million by 2030 and as high as 16 million by 2050.

Overview

66With some illnesses you can still live and love with your mind intact; with Alzheimer's you lose abstract thought, reasoning, and judgment. People fear this more than cancer or heart disease.99

—Dr. Howard Fillit, quoted in Diane Guernsey, "What You Need to Know About Alzheimer's."

66Alzheimer's disease is an octopus. Its tentacles stretch out through the ether, strangling the lives of those within its reach. The aftermath . . . leaves survivors weaving the frayed threads of their lives into lessons colored in grief, anger, fear, sadness, and human frailty.99

—Ihla Nation, "Alzheimer's, Artichokes, and Forgiveness."

On November 5, 1994, a letter written by former president Ronald Reagan was released to the public. Reagan had just been diagnosed with Alzheimer's disease. Rather than keep it a private family matter, he decided to share the news with the American people in order to promote greater awareness of the disease. "Perhaps it will encourage a clearer understanding of the individuals and families who are affected by it," he wrote. Reagan acknowledged that as time went by, his family would undoubtedly bear a heavy burden and he wished that he could spare them from that. He added that he planned to live the remainder of his life doing things he had always enjoyed and to stay in touch with his friends and supporters. His letter ended with a heartfelt conclusion:

In closing let me thank you, the American people for giving me the great honor of allowing me to serve as your President. When the Lord calls me home, whenever that may be I will face it with the greatest love for this country of ours and eternal optimism for its future. I now begin the journey that will lead me into the sunset of my life. I know that for America there will always be a bright dawn ahead.[1]

Reagan's condition began to deteriorate, and 10 years later he died from Alzheimer's-related complications.

Although many people were saddened by Reagan's death, some good resulted from it because, as he had wished, his struggle with the disease created greater awareness of Alzheimer's. Today Alzheimer's research is being aggressively pursued, and far more is known about the disease than a decade ago. Still, however, Alzheimer's continues to plague millions of people and has escalated into what scientists and advocacy organizations are calling a public health crisis. According to a 2008 report by the Centers for Disease Control and Prevention (CDC), in 2005 Alzheimer's disease was the seventh-leading cause of death for people of all ages and the fifth-leading cause of death for people aged 65 and older. Clearly, as far as research has progressed, still much more work remains.

> " Alzheimer's is a progressive, irreversible, and fatal disease of the brain. "

What Is Alzheimer's Disease?

Alzheimer's is a progressive, irreversible, and fatal disease of the brain. It is part of a family of diseases known as dementia, meaning "deprived of mind," which is the general term for loss of memory and other cognitive abilities that is serious enough to interfere with daily life. Of the different forms of dementia that exist, Alzheimer's comprises 60 to 80 percent of all cases. The 2 types of Alzheimer's are late-onset, which occurs after the age of 65 and is by far the most common; and early-onset, which is extremely rare and occurs in less than 5 percent of all Alzheimer's cases. Early-onset Alzheimer's develops before age 65 and can affect people in their thirties and forties. In December 2007 Terry Pratchett, a well-known British science-fiction author, publicly announced that he had been diagnosed with a very rare form of early-onset Alzheimer's known as posterior cortical atrophy. As shocking as the news was, Pratchett vowed to do everything possible to fight the disease, and he even faced it with his trademark sense of humor. In a letter he posted online titled "An Embuggerance," he asked people to remain optimistic about his prognosis:

> I would just like to draw attention to everyone reading the above that this should be interpreted as "I am not dead." I will, of course, be dead at some future point, as will everybody else. For me, this may be further off than you think—it's too soon to tell. I know it's a very human thing to say "Is there anything I can do," but in this case I would only entertain offers from very high-end experts in brain chemistry.[2]

One of the greatest myths about Alzheimer's is that it is a normal part of aging. Although it is true that people's memories are often not as sharp as they get older, the memory loss in Alzheimer's patients is abnormal and severe. Rudolph Tanzi, a professor of neurology at Harvard University Medical School whose primary specialty is Alzheimer's research, explains:

> Think of your brain as a stereo whose music is memory. Your stereo works great for a lot of years. Eventually, as it ages, it occasionally short circuits. That's normal decline, normal wear and tear. In Alzheimer's, there's a toxic invader in the stereo—one that actively destroys the wires that make up the circuit. It doesn't just temporarily disrupt the music, it silences it.[3]

How Does Alzheimer's Disease Affect the Brain?

Alzheimer's disease attacks the brain, literally causing it to waste away. Yet exactly why this happens is still a mystery, as the Alzheimer's Association states: "Scientists do not yet fully understand the processes resulting in the catastrophic brain damage associated with Alzheimer's disease."[4] What scientists do know is that the brains of people with Alzheimer's become clogged up with two abnormal structures known as beta-amyloid

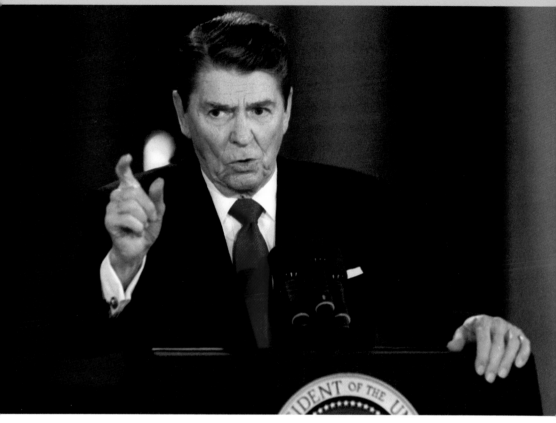

Former president Ronald Reagan revealed in 1994 that he was suffering from Alzheimer's disease. He chose to share the news with the American people in order to promote greater awareness of the disease. Reagan succumbed to the disease on June 5, 2004.

plaques and neurofibrillary tangles. Plaques are tiny, insoluble (not dissolvable) fragments of protein and cellular material that build up outside and around neurons, or nerve cells in the brain. Scientists have compared plaques to tiny Brillo pads. Tangles are insoluble, twisted fibers that build up inside dead and dying neurons. Although researchers are not exactly sure what role plaques and tangles play in Alzheimer's disease, they believe that nerve cell communication somehow becomes blocked, disrupting activities that the cells need to survive. This disruption causes neurons to stop working and lose their connections with other neurons, which leads to memory failure and other problems.

Over time, the brain becomes so filled with plaques and tangles that it atrophies, or shrinks, and eventually the cells die, leading to the death of the patient. The time from diagnosis to death can vary from just a few years to 10 or more years, usually depending on how old the patient is when diagnosed and how far the brain damage has progressed. Most people with Alzheimer's die from other illnesses, such as aspiration pneumonia, which occurs when they inadvertently breathe food or liquid into their lungs because they lose their ability to swallow; malnutrition; or infection. Stephen Henderson's father forgot how to swallow properly, causing saliva to collect in his lungs. This led to the severe infection that eventually killed him.

What Causes Alzheimer's Disease?

Although the effects of Alzheimer's are well understood, scientists do not know what causes the disease. It is not like diseases such as diphtheria, polio, or measles, all of which have clear-cut causes and can be prevented with vaccinations or cured with antibiotics. According to the National Institute on Aging (NIA) Alzheimer's is more similar to diabetes or arthritis, which develop due to a combination of genetics, lifestyle, and environmental factors that work together to cause the onset of the diseases. Research has shown that people who have other illnesses, such as cardiovascular disease, high blood pressure, diabetes, or high cholesterol, have a potentially greater risk of developing Alzheimer's. By far, though, the greatest risk factor for Alzheimer's is advancing age. Every five years beyond the age of 65, someone's risk for developing the disease doubles.

> " A study led by researchers at the Johns Hopkins Bloomberg School of Public Health concluded that more than 26 million people worldwide were living with Alzheimer's in 2006. "

Who Suffers from Alzheimer's Disease?

Tens of millions of people throughout the world have been diagnosed with Alzheimer's. A study led by researchers at the Johns Hopkins Bloomberg School of Public Health concluded that more than 26 million people worldwide were living with Alzheimer's in 2006. In the United States, an estimated 5.2 million people have the disease, which is a 10 percent increase since 2002. Because of the steady growth in the older population, the prevalence of Alzheimer's continues to increase every year and is expected to skyrocket in the future. The Alzheimer's Association explains:

> In 2000, there were an estimated 411,000 new cases of Alzheimer's disease [in the United States]. That number is expected to increase to 454,000 new cases a year by 2010, 615,000 new cases a year by 2030, and 959,000 new cases a year by 2050. . . . By 2050, the number of individuals age 65 and over with Alzheimer's could range from 11 million to 16 million unless science finds a way to prevent or effectively treat the disease. By that date, more than 60 percent of people with Alzheimer's disease will be age 85 or older.[5]

The Stages of Alzheimer's Disease

Although the progression of Alzheimer's varies from patient to patient, symptoms of the disease tend to develop over the same typical stages. The earliest phase, known as preclinical Alzheimer's, is a time when memory loss seems to be greater than what is normal for someone's particular age, but it may not be obvious to family, friends, or even the person's physician. As the brain continues to atrophy, the presence of Alzheimer's becomes more obvious. Memory loss grows worse, and patients make repetitive statements and ask the same questions over and over because they do not remember having asked them. They often misplace things and forget where they put them. Kali Van Baale, whose husband suffered from Alzheimer's, recalls one occasion when she was helping him hunt for his glasses. She found that he had put his T-shirt in the toilet, the remote control in the microwave oven, and had poured his morning coffee into the sugar bowl. Equally as common as forgetfulness are personality changes and mood swings. Ruth A. Brandwein began noticing radical changes in her mother's personality, and she suspected some type of dementia. She writes:

> Mom began to be paranoid, imagining her neighbors breaking into her home and stealing old clothes from the basement. At first, we wanted to believe her. . . . But final-

ly, when she insisted that a neighbor had climbed through the window to steal the electric bill that she couldn't find, we had the doctor assess her condition. She confirmed that Mom was in the early stages of Alzheimer's.[6]

In the moderate stage of Alzheimer's, memory loss becomes much more pronounced, and this can be extremely frustrating for patients. Richard Taylor, a retired psychologist who was diagnosed with Alzheimer's disease at the age of 58, shares a poignant analogy from the viewpoint of someone who has lived through it:

> Sometimes, when I am alone with my thoughts, I wander aimlessly around the corridors of my mind. I open various doors to see if they are still full of the memories I stored there long ago. To my pleasant surprise, most of them seem to contain all that I remember putting in the room. However, as I move from the past toward the present, I find more and more empty rooms. Not only are they empty, they are dark. They offer no clue, other than the label on the door, as to what they once contained. . . . It is very unnerving to be in the midst of a conversation and all of a sudden need to open the door to a room to access its contents and—the room is dark.[7]

Also in the moderate phase, people often become confused and disoriented and have a tendency to wander away from familiar surroundings and get lost. They have problems recognizing their friends and family and have difficulty organizing thoughts, reading, writing, and even speaking. They lack the ability to learn new things or cope with unexpected situations. They become easily agitated; exhibit inappropriate behavior, such as throwing food at family members, kicking, or hitting; and are prone to outbursts of vulgar language. A common behavior is for

> **Alzheimer's disease attacks the brain, literally causing it to waste away. Yet exactly why this happens is still a mystery.**

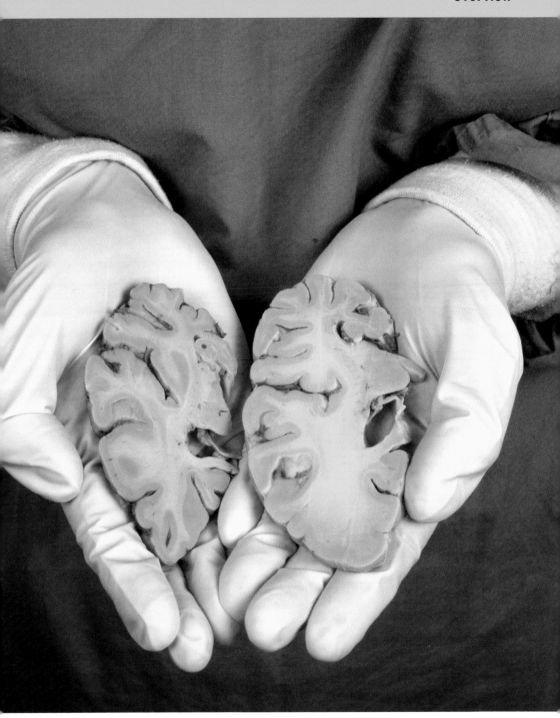

These brain samples show the physical differences Alzheimer's disease can have on the brain. The shrunken sample on the left is an Alzheimer's-diseased slice, the sample on the right is from a healthy brain.

patients to become increasingly agitated, confused, and restless toward the end of the day, which is known as sundowning.

In the advanced, most severe stage, the disease has progressed so far that Alzheimer's patients no longer even resemble the people they once were. The NIA explains the severity of this phase of the disease: "In the last stage of AD, plaques and tangles are widespread throughout the brain, and areas of the brain have atrophied further. Patients cannot recognize family and loved ones or communicate in any way. They are completely dependent on others for care. All sense of self seems to vanish."[8] At this point, death is likely not far off.

How Alzheimer's Disease Is Diagnosed

In the past, the only way scientists could tell if someone had Alzheimer's disease was to actually see the plaques and tangles in the brain, which was only possible after the patient had died and an autopsy was performed. Today Alzheimer's can be diagnosed while someone is alive, although diagnoses are still limited to "possible" or "probable," rather than being absolute. According to the National Institutes of Health (NIH), however, at specialized medical facilities Alzheimer's can be diagnosed correctly as much as 90 percent of the time. Physicians give patients tests of memory, problem solving, attention, counting, and language. They may also perform medical tests that measure blood, spinal fluid, or urine chemistry, which can show abnormalities and possibly indicate the progression of Alzheimer's.

Sophisticated technology is also improving physicians' ability to diagnose Alzheimer's disease. For example, magnetic resonance imaging (MRI) can show abnormal shrinking of the brain, and positron-emission tomography (PET), an imaging technique that allows researchers to observe and measure activity in various parts of the brain, can detect the presence of plaques. Both of these diagnostic tools provide windows into the living brain and can help with measuring how far the disease has progressed.

Can Lifestyle Changes Prevent or Delay Alzheimer's?

Because so much is still unknown about Alzheimer's disease, prevention cannot be guaranteed. But researchers continue to explore the positive differences that can be made when people engage in healthy lifestyles and do everything possible to maintain good brain health. One factor that was identified years ago is the connection between cardiovascular health and the condition of the brain. The results of a 20-year study involving 469 senior citizens in the Bronx section of New York City were published in 2003. The research showed that elderly women who previously had heart attacks were 5 times more likely to develop Alzheimer's disease or other forms of dementia than other women of the same age. A different study, published in 2005, showed that people with three or more cardiovascular risk factors (such as high blood pressure, diabetes, and smoking) were more likely to develop Alzheimer's than people without such risk factors. People who exercise regularly and keep physically fit are also thought to have a lower risk of developing the disease.

Research has also shown that people who keep their brains active by doing mentally challenging activities have a lower tendency of developing Alzheimer's later in life. In the Bronx study, researchers found that playing chess or bridge, reading, playing a musical instrument, or doing crossword puzzles, significantly lowered the risk of someone developing dementia. The researchers noted that the participants who played board games had a 74 percent lower risk for dementia, those who played an instrument had a 69 percent lower risk, and those who did crossword puzzles at least 4 days a week lowered their risk by 47 percent. Joseph Coyle, a professor of psychiatry and neuroscience at Harvard Medical School, says that neuroscientists are finding that the brain has "plasticity," meaning that thoughts and experiences may change neural structure and brain chemistry. He explains: "Using the mind actually causes rewiring of the brain, sprouting new synapses—it may even cause the generation of new neurons. So psychology trumps biology."[9]

> " Today Alzheimer's can be diagnosed while someone is alive, although diagnoses are still limited to 'possible' or 'probable,' rather than being absolute. "

How Is Alzheimer's Treated?

Alzheimer's cannot be cured, nor can the deterioration and death of brain cells be stopped. As with any disease, however, the earlier it is discovered, the more effective treatment may be. Some drugs have been shown to slow the progression of Alzheimer's and, in the process, help with cognitive symptoms. As the Madison Institute of Medicine writes, "In the past, medications were thought to offer very little to patients with Alzheimer's disease. This is no longer true. Unfortunately, some people who write about Alzheimer's disease still hold these outdated beliefs, ignoring the sound research that supports the use of medications."[10] One group of drugs that may be prescribed for Alzheimer's patients is cholinesterase inhibitors. Scientists have learned that a dramatic drop in the level of a chemical known as acetylcholine, a chemical that transmits messages in the brain, occurs in the brains of people with Alzheimer's. Acetylcholine is rapidly broken down by an enzyme called acetylcholinesterase, which results in a disruption of message transmission and adversely affects attention and memory. According to the Mayo Clinic, the enzyme can be blocked with cholinesterase inhibitors, which could help improve cognitive and neuropsychiatric symptoms and possibly have an effect on the long-term course of the disease.

> **During this [advanced Alzheimer's] phase, patients often regress to a childlike state, and playing with toys or having someone read to them is comforting.**

At some nursing homes, caregivers use an unusual approach to help Alzheimer's patients improve their memory: children's toys, games, and picture books. Their reasoning is that in late-stage Alzheimer's, most of the brain has deteriorated except the area that controls senses and motor function. During this phase, patients often regress to a childlike state, and playing with toys or having someone read to them is comforting. Games that teach children how to tie shoes, zip coats, and unbutton pockets can help strengthen skills and restore confidence to patients. For those who have lost their memories, playing with dolls can possibly rekindle thoughts of raising children as well as allow them to show affection. Miriam Josef, a social worker at a hospice in New York, explains: "As people move toward the end of life and start to regress, they go back to childhood. Toys soothe children. Why wouldn't they soothe those with dementia?"[11]

Will Research Prevent or Cure Alzheimer's Disease?

As researchers continue to study Alzheimer's, they are making exciting discoveries that could potentially lead to preventive treatments as well as new drugs that could slow the disease's progression and possibly cure people who suffer from it. A team of scientists from Scotland announced in July 2007 that they had developed a chemical that prevented Alzheimer's from killing brain cells in mice. Researchers from Zurich, Switzerland, have been working to perfect a vaccination that could potentially stop the progression of Alzheimer's by breaking up plaques in the brain. At the University of California, San Diego, researchers are working on a type of therapy that involves genetically modifying skin cells and injecting them into the brains of Alzheimer's patients, which will hopefully repair damage to neurons and prompt the growth of new, healthy ones. Andy Dillin, a scientist with the Salk Institute in La Jolla, California, has identified a gene that extends the lives of worms—and makes them immune to Alzheimer's disease. These are just a few of the research breakthroughs that scientists have been making, and many others are under way. The NIA explains why these achievements are so promising: "Results from this research will bring us closer to the day when we will be able to prevent or even cure the devastating disease that robs our older relatives and friends of their most precious possession—their minds."[12]

How Does Alzheimer's Disease Affect the Brain?

> 66Alzheimer's disease will kill you.... It slowly and painful-ly takes away your identity, ability to connect with oth-ers, think, eat, talk, walk and find your way home.99
>
> —Alzheimer's Association, "Alzheimer Myths."

> 66The terrible thing about Alzheimer's is . . . it robs the victim of the memories, the tapestry of memories and recollections that constitute the self in so many ways, and not only does the victim lose their own sense of self . . . but the people around them, the loved ones, begin to question whether this is the same person we always knew.99
>
> —Ron Reagan, son of Ronald Reagan, in PBS's *Online NewsHour* special "Stealing Minds."

In 1901 a German physician named Alois Alzheimer consulted with Auguste Deter, a 51-year-old woman who was admitted to a hospital in Frankfurt, Germany, after exhibiting strange behavior. According to her family, Deter was suffering from memory problems, disorienta-tion, and paranoia. She had been hiding objects in her home and was experiencing strong feelings of jealousy toward her husband, unjustly believing him to be unfaithful. Alzheimer later wrote that when he first saw the woman lying in a hospital bed, she had a helpless expression on her face. In talking with her he found that she remembered her own name, but not her husband's name; in fact, she became confused when asked if she was married. She did not know how long she had been in the hospital, and when asked what year it was, she replied that it was 1800. When Alzheimer showed her a purse, a key, a pencil, a diary, a book, and a cigar, she identified the objects correctly but soon forgot what had been shown to her. When she ate cauliflower and pork for lunch, she told Alzheimer that she was eating spinach. As she chewed meat and was asked what she was doing, she answered that she was eating potatoes and horseradish.

> " **[Alzheimer] discovered dramatic shrinkage as well as microscopic deposits that he had never seen before: abnormal clumps (plaques) and tangled bundles of fibers (tangles).** "

Over the following years, Deter's condition continued to deteriorate. She lost cognitive functions, suffered from hallucinations, and was haunted by irrational fears. Eventually she was bedridden and mute, and in April 1906 she died at the age of 55. After her death, Alzheimer, who had moved to Munich in 1903, asked that Deter's brain be sent to him so he could closely examine it. He discovered dramatic shrinkage as well as microscopic deposits that he had never seen before: abnormal clumps (plaques) and twisted bundles of hairlike fibers (tangles). Alzheimer spoke of his discoveries about "Frau Auguste D." at a lecture presented in Tübingen, Germany, on November 4, 1906. One year later, he published his lecture under the title, "A Characteristic Serious Disease of the Cerebral Cortex," in which he stated that "all in all we have to face a peculiar disease process. Such peculiar disease processes have been verified recently in considerable numbers."[13]

Brain Function and Deterioration

The human brain weighs only 3 or 4 pounds (1.4 or 1.8kg), but it is a highly complex and powerful organ. The largest section is composed of 2 hemispheres (also called the cerebrum), which account for 85 percent of the brain's weight and are connected by a thick bundle of nerves called the corpus callosum. The left hemisphere is thought to control speech, writing, language, and calculation, and the right hemisphere is involved in spatial abilities, visual face recognition, and creativity. The 2 hemispheres are surrounded by an outer layer called the cerebral cortex, which is where the brain processes sensory information from the outside world and controls perception, emotion, conscious thought, planning, and decision making. Deep within the cerebrum is the hippocampus, which is important for learning and short-term memory and is thought to be the area where short-term memories are converted into long-term memories that are stored in other parts of the brain. The brain stem, located at the base of the brain, forms a connection with the spinal cord and controls heart rate, blood pressure, and breathing and influences sleep and dreaming. In the back of the head, between the cerebrum and brain stem, is the cerebellum, which comprises about 10 percent of the brain and is responsible for the coordination of movement and balance. The cerebellum also has 2 hemispheres, and the NIA explains their importance:

> **Groups of nerve cells have their own specialized jobs. Some are involved in thinking, learning, and memory, and others tell muscles when and how to move.**

> They are always receiving information from the eyes, ears, and muscles and joints about the body's movements and position. Once the cerebellum processes the information, it works through the rest of the brain and spinal cord to send out instructions to the body. The cerebellum's work allows us to walk smoothly, maintain our balance, and turn around without even thinking about it.[14]

Within the various sections of the brain are approximately 100 billion nerve cells, or neurons. These neurons have the ability to gather and transmit electrochemical signals to each other across tiny gaps between them known as synapses. Groups of nerve cells have their own specialized jobs. Some are involved in thinking, learning, and memory, and others tell muscles when and how to move. The Alzheimer's Association uses an analogy to explain how the neurons operate: "To do their work, brain cells operate like tiny factories. They receive supplies, generate energy, construct equipment and get rid of waste. Cells also process and store information and communicate with other cells. Keeping everything running requires coordination as well as large amounts of fuel and oxygen." Continuing with the factory analogy, scientists believe that Alzheimer's disease prevents part of a cell's "factory" from running well, as the Alzheimer's Association states: "They are not sure where the trouble starts. But just like a real factory, backups and breakdowns in one system cause problems in other areas. As damage spreads, cells lose their ability to do their jobs and, eventually, die."[15]

Insidious Plaques and Tangles

Once Alzheimer's disease has set in, plaques begin to develop in certain areas of the brain. In a study that was published in February 2008, researchers from Massachusetts reported that plaques could develop in just 24 hours, and nerve cell changes began to appear within days. Although scientists do not know what triggers the formation of plaques, they have a good understanding of how they form. A gene known as the APP gene provides the brain with instructions for making a protein called amyloid precursor protein, which is located in many different tissues and organs, including the brain and spinal cord. Within individual cells, the protein is divided into small fragments by enzymes. Scientists believe that amyloid helps neurons grow and survive and may aid in the repair of damaged neurons.

> " As plaques continue to build up, tau proteins undergo chemical changes that cause them to bundle together and form tangles inside dead and dying neurons. "

In brains affected by Alzheimer's disease, however, some fragments that break off from the amyloid precursor protein mysteriously change shape, become extremely sticky, and fuse together with molecules, neurons, and nonnerve cells. This leads to the formation of clumps between and around neurons, known as plaques. According to the Mayo Clinic, these plaques are similar to the substance that clogs heart arteries. Sam Gandy, who is a neuroscientist and the chief scientific adviser to the Alzheimer's Association, describes this formation: "The process that begins Alzheimer's disease is what we call protein folding, and literally the amyloid protein folds back on itself like a big bobby-pin. And this then is a sticky form, and many of these bobby pin-like sticky structures aggregate together, clump together."[16] Scientists do not know if plaques cause Alzheimer's or whether they are possibly a by-product of the disease process.

> As Alzheimer's progresses to its advanced stages, patients often lose their memories entirely, are unable to recognize family and friends, forget who they are, and lose their ability to communicate or interact at all.

Healthy neurons have internal scaffoldlike structures (known as microtubules) that serve as pathways along which information travels throughout the brain. These microtubules are strengthened and stabilized by a protein known as tau—but in brains affected by Alzheimer's disease, the role of tau becomes destructive. As plaques continue to build up, tau proteins undergo chemical changes that cause them to bundle together and form tangles inside dead and dying neurons. This leads to the collapse of the neuron's support structures, destroying the pathways along which information travels through the brain. The Mayo Clinic explains: "As Alzheimer's develops, the shape of tau molecules inside neurons changes; the molecules begin to fall off the microtubules they once supported, and bind to form paired and twisted filaments. The process is toxic to the microtubules, which can no longer transport the molecular cargo needed to keep the neuron alive."[17] As neurons continue to die, fewer are available for information storage and retrieval, which results first in malfunctions in memory and later in the more severe symptoms of Alzheimer's.

How the Damage Spreads

Scientists believe that plaques first begin to develop in the entorhinal cortex, an area of the brain that is near the hippocampus and has direct connections to it. As plaques multiply and tangles start to form, these abnormal structures spread to the hippocampus, which is essential for the formation of short- and long-term memories. Along the way affected regions start to atrophy and memory begins to fail. As plaques and tangles move into the cerebral cortex, memory loss grows worse and the patient develops other cognitive problems, such as confusion, poor judgment, lack of motivation and initiative, and increased anxiety. The damage continues to spread to the areas of the cerebral cortex that control language, reasoning, sensory processing, and conscious thought. At this stage symptoms become more pronounced, and patients are prone to behavior problems, agitation, and delusions as well as severely impaired memory function.

As Alzheimer's progresses to its advanced stages, patients often lose their memories entirely, are unable to recognize family and friends, forget who they are, and lose their ability to communicate or interact at all. This is devastating for the people who love them, as Merle Comer, whose husband has Alzheimer's, explains: "Somebody once described it as a house where you see one light go off at a time, or watching somebody in slow motion die . . . literally lose their mind in front of your eyes. Very painful to watch, especially knowing what he was."[18]

"A Horrible Way to See Him"

It is painful for Ron Wheeler to talk about his father's descent into the abyss of Alzheimer's disease, which eventually took his life. Dick Wheeler served in the U.S. Navy during World War II; had a long, successful career in newspaper publishing; and was fully enjoying his retirement. Then, at age 77, his family began to notice changes that they found disturbing. "It was both his memory and his judgment," says Ron Wheeler:

> He could ride his bike all the way across town to the Buick dealership where he remembered buying his car, had vivid memories of the war and his military service, and remembered other things from long ago. But when we mentioned his friends, he would say, "Who are they?

I don't know them"—and he'd known them for years. He also bought a sporty new car on a whim and paid $2,500 for an extended warranty, which he would never, ever have done in the past. It was obvious that something was very wrong.[19]

The elder Wheeler was diagnosed with Alzheimer's, and the disease rapidly took its toll on his brain. His driving ability steadily worsened, and he often got lost in the city where he had lived his entire life, which necessitated his family getting his driver's license taken away. "That just broke his heart," says Wheeler. "He was totally crushed and he didn't understand why he couldn't drive anymore. He even rode his bike to the police station once and asked them, 'Why did you take my driver's license away? I didn't do anything wrong. I'm a good driver.' Even though we knew we didn't have a choice, we felt terrible having to do that to him." Deprived of his vehicle, the elder Wheeler took to riding his bike everywhere he wanted to go and was often gone for hours at a time. Then, on a frigid, rainy night in February 2006, Ron Wheeler got a phone call from his brother. Their dad had gone for a long bike ride and had gotten disoriented and lost. He ended up at a grocery store, freezing and soaking wet, miles away from his intended destination with no idea where he was. "After that point we had to take away his bike too," says Wheeler. "There's no way to explain how it made us feel to hurt him so badly."[20]

Based on a doctor's recommendation, the elder Wheeler was admitted to a special hospital program for dementia patients and then later was placed in a long-term care facility. Wheeler says:

He hated it there, even though I don't think he even knew where he was. He lived less than three weeks after that, and I'm convinced that he just did not want to live that way. Only a few years before, his will to live was very strong, and his body was like that of someone 25 years younger. But Alzheimer's stripped this once-strong man of his will to live. At the very end, I would look at him lying in the hospital bed and he seemed like an entirely different person. He didn't know who he was, he didn't know my mom, or my brothers, or me. It was like he wasn't even alive anymore—he was just existing, and although his body was still strong, his brain had wasted away and his mind was gone. It was a horrible way to see him.[21]

Wheeler says that unlike many Alzheimer's sufferers, his father never seemed angry, was not prone to outbursts, and never exhibited inappropriate language or behavior, as he explains:

> He just seemed sad; so very sad, lonely, and confused about why people were taking things away from him and why he couldn't go home. All he wanted to do was to go home, and we couldn't let him because we were afraid if our mom kept trying to care for him, we would lose her too. For anyone who hasn't lived through such an awful experience with someone they love, they just cannot imagine what it's like.[22]

Still a Mystery

There is no denying that Alzheimer's is a tragic, devastating disease. Once plaques and tangles start to form and spread, they clog up the brain and destroy it by damaging and killing nerve cells. Scientists desperately search for a better understanding of why these abnormal structures form in the first place and whether they cause Alzheimer's or are merely by-products of it. If research can provide answers to those questions and others, perhaps Alzheimer's disease will someday be a thing of the past rather than a death sentence for everyone who suffers from it.

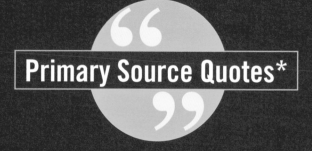

Primary Source Quotes*

How Does Alzheimer's Disease Affect the Brain?

❝The cruelty of Alzheimer's disease is that it attacks the brain, profoundly altering who we are.❞

—Fisher Center for Alzheimer's Research Foundation, "Alzheimer's Disease Cause, Care, and Cure," 2008. www.alzinfo.org.

The Fisher Center for Alzheimer's Research Foundation funds more than 85 scientists throughout the United States in search of a cure for Alzheimer's disease.

❝As the disease progresses, it's on a malignant process. It destroys not only the nerve cells in the hippocampus responsible for memory, but many of the cells throughout the top of the brain, called the cortex. This is the master circuitry of the brain.❞

—Sam Gandy, "Families Advocate for Alzheimer's Disease to Be National Priority," *PBS Online NewsHour*, July 26, 2006. www.pbs.org.

Gandy is a neuroscientist at Thomas Jefferson University and is the chief scientific adviser to the Alzheimer's Association.

* Editor's Note: While the definition of a primary source can be narrowly or broadly defined, for the purposes of Compact Research, a primary source consists of: 1) results of original research presented by an organization or researcher; 2) eyewitness accounts of events, personal experience, or work experience; 3) first-person editorials offering pundits' opinions; 4) government officials presenting political plans and/or policies; 5) representatives of organizations presenting testimony or policy.

66 **The essential nature of Alzheimer's disease—losing your mind—terrifies everyone who has seen a friend or family member fall to its advance.** 99

—Vernon M. Ingram, "Alzheimer's Disease," *American Scientist*, July/August 2003. www.americanscientist.org.

Ingram is a professor of biology at the Massachusetts Institute of Technology.

66 **So much is lost when Alzheimer's claims someone. Memory is only one of the casualties. The days and years you thought you'd have with your loved one fall by the wayside, the conversations you always dreamed of having must be put away, relinquished.** 99

—Patti Davis, "Letting Go," *Newsweek*, November 14, 2007. www.newsweek.com.

Davis is the daughter of Ronald Reagan, former president of the United States who died of Alzheimer's disease in June 2004.

66 **The disease works slowly, destroying the mind, stealing life in a tedious, silent dance of death.** 99

—Thomas DeBaggio, *Losing My Mind: An Intimate Look at Life with Alzheimer's.* New York: Free Press, 2002.

DeBaggio was diagnosed with early-onset Alzheimer's at the age of 57, and he wrote a book about his experience as the disease progressed.

66 **Alzheimer's disease is a progressive, irreversible brain disorder with no known cause or cure. It attacks and slowly steals the minds of its victims.** 99

—American Health Assistance Foundation, "Alzheimer's Disease: About Alzheimer's," 2007. www.ahaf.org.

The American Health Assistance Foundation is a nonprofit organization that funds research into cures for Alzheimer's and other diseases.

❝Alzheimer's is not a disease so much as it is a tragedy. . . . Death comes with aching slowness and leaves, in its wake, utter devastation.❞

—Kate Mulgrew, "Keynote Speech," Alzheimer's Women's Auxiliary for Research and Education, November 3, 2005. www.totallykate.com.

Mulgrew is an actress and writer whose mother died of Alzheimer's disease in 2006.

❝The formation of amyloid plaques and neurofibrillary tangles are thought to contribute to the degradation of the neurons (nerve cells) in the brain and the subsequent symptoms of Alzheimer's disease.❞

—American Health Assistance Foundation, "Amyloid Plaques and Neurofibrillary Tangles," February 14, 2007. www.ahaf.org.

The American Health Assistance Foundation funds research that seeks cures for Alzheimer's and other diseases and provides the public with information about risk factors, preventive lifestyles, and available treatments.

❝Although plaques and tangles are the conventionally accepted perpetrators of Alzheimer's, their respective roles remain controversial and there is a question of whether there is enough evidence to implicate them as causal agents in [Alzheimer's disease].❞

—Peter J. Whitehouse, *The Myth of Alzheimer's*. New York: St. Martin's, 2008.

Whitehouse is a neurologist who specializes in geriatrics and cognitive science, with a focus on dementia.

❝Alzheimer's disease is a process in which brain cells deteriorate and die. This process ('neurodegeneration') likely goes on over many years before sufficient brain cells are damaged such that brain functions fail and symptoms of brain failure emerge.❞

—John C. Morris, "Readers' Questions: Alzheimer's Disease," *New York Times*, December 26, 2007. http://science.blogs.nytimes.com.

Morris is director of the Alzheimer's disease research center at Washington University in St. Louis.

❝In my view, [Alzheimer's disease] pathology represents one of the most severe of a long list of factors that simply degrade the ability of the brain to translate what it sees, hears, feels, smells and tastes in actions crucial for controlling thought and action and self-reference.❞

—Michael Merzenich, "A Sixth Misconception About Aging," *On the Brain*, May 13, 2008. http://merzenich.positscience.com.

Merzenich is a scientist and educator as well as the founder of the Scientific Learning Corporation and Neuroscience Solutions Corporation in California.

❝Although seizures are not a common symptom of Alzheimer's disease (AD), the brains of people with AD could be humming with seizure-like activity, interrupted by quiet rebound periods that do more harm than good.❞

—National Institute of Neurological Disorders and Stroke (NINDS), "A Roller Coaster of Seizure-Like Activity May Damage the Alzheimer's Brain," November 27, 2007. www.ninds.nih.gov.

The NINDS seeks to reduce the burden of neurological disease suffered by people all over the world.

How Does Alzheimer's Disease Affect the Brain?

- Alzheimer's disease occurs in an estimated **60 to 80 percent** of all dementia cases.

- Dementias **other than Alzheimer's** include vascular dementia, mixed dementia, dementia with Lewy bodies, frontotemporal dementia (including Pick's disease), Creutzfeldt-Jakob disease, and normal pressure hydrocephalus.

- In 2005 Alzheimer's claimed the lives of nearly **72,000** people—up from 14,112 in 1991.

- Autopsy studies show that most people develop some **plaques and tangles** in the brain as they age, but those with Alzheimer's develop far more than what is normal.

- Alzheimer's causes brain cells to **lose their ability to form new connections** with other cells, causing the information stored within them to fade away.

- The Alzheimer's Association states that **60 percent** of people with Alzheimer's will wander and become lost.

- In Alzheimer's most advanced stages, there is dramatic **shrinkage in the brain** from cell loss as well as widespread debris from dead and dying neurons.

The Brain and Its Functions

The human brain weighs only about three pounds, but it is a complex, powerful organ that controls everything from breathing and blood pressure to memory, thought processing, and movement. This illustration shows the major segments of a normal brain and their various functions before the brain has been invaded by Alzheimer's disease.

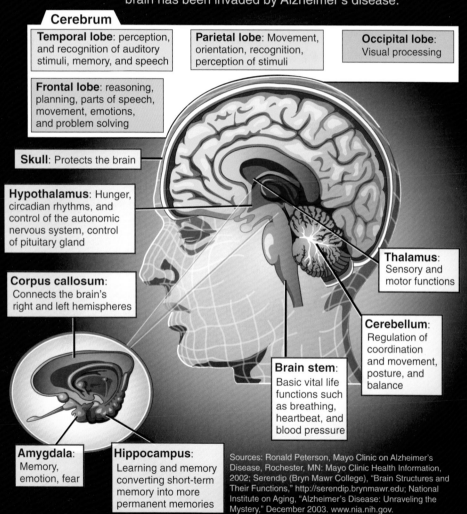

Cerebrum

Temporal lobe: perception, and recognition of auditory stimuli, memory, and speech

Parietal lobe: Movement, orientation, recognition, perception of stimuli

Occipital lobe: Visual processing

Frontal lobe: reasoning, planning, parts of speech, movement, emotions, and problem solving

Skull: Protects the brain

Hypothalamus: Hunger, circadian rhythms, and control of the autonomic nervous system, control of pituitary gland

Corpus callosum: Connects the brain's right and left hemispheres

Thalamus: Sensory and motor functions

Cerebellum: Regulation of coordination and movement, posture, and balance

Brain stem: Basic vital life functions such as breathing, heartbeat, and blood pressure

Amygdala: Memory, emotion, fear

Hippocampus: Learning and memory converting short-term memory into more permanent memories

Sources: Ronald Peterson, Mayo Clinic on Alzheimer's Disease, Rochester, MN: Mayo Clinic Health Information, 2002; Serendip (Bryn Mawr College), "Brain Structures and Their Functions," http://serendip.brynmawr.edu; National Institute on Aging, "Alzheimer's Disease: Unraveling the Mystery," December 2003. www.nia.nih.gov.

- Scientists believe that brain changes may start **10 to 20 years** before any signs or symptoms of Alzheimer's disease appear.

Alzheimer's Destroys the Brain

Although scientists do not know why it happens, Alzheimer's ravages the brain, litterally causing it to atrophy and waste away. Abnormal microscopic deposits known as plaques (a mass or buildup of proteins) and tangles (bunched up or knotted nerve cells) form and spread,until eventually brain function is lost. These illustrations show how brain and nerve cells (neurons) change as Alzheimer's disease progresses.

Preclinical Alzheimer's Disease

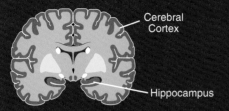

Cerebral Cortex

Hippocampus

Mild memory loss

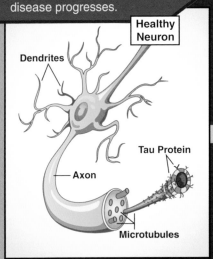

Healthy Neuron

Dendrites

Tau Protein

Axon

Microtubules

Mild Alzheimer's Disease

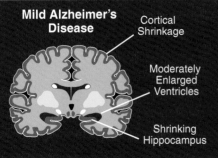

Cortical Shrinkage

Moderately Enlarged Ventricles

Shrinking Hippocampus

More serious memory loss; confusion; disorientation; poor judgement leading to bad decisions; tendency to wander and become lost; personality changes

Diseased Neuron

Amyloid Plaque

Disintegrating Microtubules

Severe Alzheimer's Disease

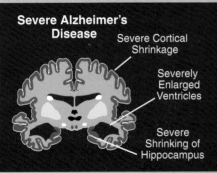

Severe Cortical Shrinkage

Severely Enlarged Ventricles

Severe Shrinking of Hippocampus

Inability to recognize friends and family; near complete loss of memory; seizures; difficulty swallowing; lack of bladder and bowel control

Sources: American Health Assistance Foundation, "How the Brain and Nerve Cells Change During Alzheimer's Disease," February 14, 2007. www.ahaf.org; National Institute on Aging, "Alzheimer's Disease: Unraveling the Mystery," December 2003. www.nia.nih.gov.

Normal Brain Aging Versus Alzheimer's-Diseased Brain

As people get older, changes occur in all parts of their bodies, including the brain. According to the National Institute on Aging, some neurons shrink, especially large ones involved in learning, memory, planning, and other complex mental activities. Plaques and tangles may also develop in the brain, although healthy people develop far fewer of them than those with Alzheimer's. These illustrations of positron emission tomography (PET) scans show differences between the brain of a healthy 20-year-old, a normal 80-year-old, and someone whose brain has been ravaged by Alzheimer's disease.

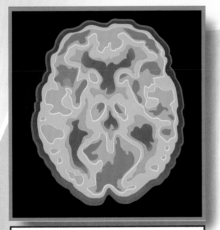

PET scan of healthy 20-year-old

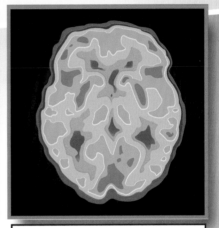

PET scan of normal 80-year-old

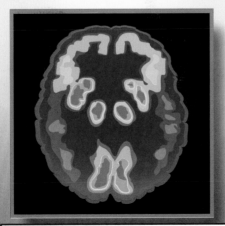

PET scan of Alzheimer's brain deteriorated by plaques and tangles.

Source: National Institute on Aging, "Alzheimer's Disease: Unraveling the Mystery," 2003. www.nia.nih.gov.

Increasing Deaths from Alzheimer's

One of the most tragic facts about Alzheimer's is that its relentless attack on the brain always leads to death. The number of people who have died from Alzheimer's disease has steadily risen since the 1990s. This increase is because people are living longer than ever before and the risk of developing Alzheimer's increases with age.

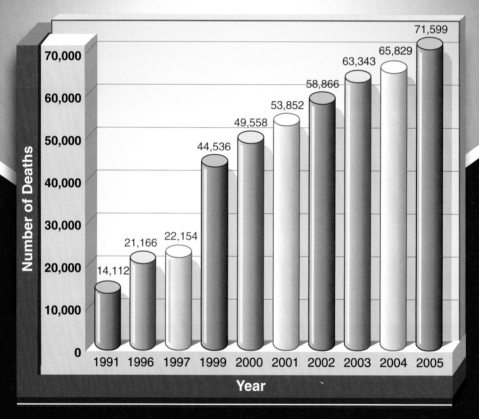

Source: Centers for Disease Control and Prevention, "Alzheimer's Deaths," 2008. www.cdc.gov.

- Studies based on autopsies of Down syndrome patients who had Alzheimer's suggest that plaques may begin to form years before symptoms of the disease appear and possibly even during **childhood**.

- In its latest stages, Alzheimer's disease **destroys brain cells** that control moving and swallowing.

What Causes Alzheimer's Disease?

66No one knows exactly what causes the Alzheimer's disease process to begin or why some of the normal changes associated with aging become so much more extreme and destructive in patients with the disease.99

—National Institute on Aging, "Alzheimer's Disease: Unraveling the Mystery."

66The key of course is to find the cause. And as of now, no one knows exactly why Alzheimer's happens. Some doctors say it's genetic, some say it's lifestyle . . . others say it's both.99

—Sanjay Gupta, "Alzheimer's Advances."

Researchers have identified distinct causes for numerous diseases. They know, for example, that influenza is caused by three strains of viruses, and malaria is a parasitic infection that is spread by the bite of certain mosquitoes. Smallpox, the only disease that has been eradicated throughout the world, originates with the variola virus. Many other diseases are also well understood, which is why they can now be prevented with vaccinations or cured with antibiotics or other medicines. Alzheimer's, however, is nothing like any of those diseases. Its cause is still unknown, so it cannot be prevented or cured. Why the brain deteriorates, why plaques and tangles form and spread, and why some people develop Alzheimer's while others do not are topics of mystery for scientists and health care professionals. That is why much of the current research focuses on finding the cause. Until the exact cause (or causes) of Alzheimer's is known, ways of preventing or curing the disease will remain elusive.

The Aging Population

Scientists may not always share the same theories about what causes Alzheimer's, but they agree on one point: Age, by far, is the greatest risk factor for developing the disease. Of the 5.2 million people who suffer from Alzheimer's in the United States, an estimated 5 million are over age 65 and 200,000 are younger. According to the Alzheimer's Association, the likelihood of people developing Alzheimer's doubles every five years after they turn 65. By the time someone has reached the age of 85, his or her chance of being stricken with the disease has risen to nearly 50 percent.

As grim as the current statistics are, the future looks even bleaker. Because of medical advancements, people now live longer than ever before, often surviving well into their eighties or nineties—which means the incidence of Alzheimer's and other dementias is expected to rise dramatically in the coming years. The Alzheimer's Association predicts that by the year 2030, the number of people aged 65 and older with the disease will reach 7.7 million—more than a 50 percent increase over today. Unless scientists find a way to prevent or cure Alzheimer's, or at least delay its onset, the number of people 65 and older with the disease could soar to 16 million by 2050. "Basically, it will approach plague proportions," says Jeffrey Cummings, director of the Alzheimer's Research Center at the University of California, Los Angeles. "Clearly we must develop a way of treating or preventing the disease because the consequences are almost unimaginable."[23]

The Role of Genetics

The more scientists learn about Alzheimer's disease, the more they become convinced that genes play a significant role in its development. Because of that, genes are the focus of numerous studies, as the Mayo Clinic explains: "Much of the research on Alzheimer's has been and remains focused on the genetic factors surrounding the disease. . . . A greater understanding has been gained from this genetic research and is providing valuable insight into the complex cascade of events that forms the disease process."[24]

In order to grasp the importance of gene studies, it is necessary to understand what genes are and the crucial role that they play. The human body is made up of trillions of microscopic cells. Within the nucleus of each cell are 23 pairs of threadlike structures known as chromosomes, which are composed of tightly coiled strands of deoxyribonucleic acid (DNA). The DNA in chromosomes is arranged into short segments called genes, whose function is to instruct cells how to produce their various proteins. The NIA explains the significance: "Genes direct almost every aspect of the construction, operation, and repair of all living things. For example, genes contain information that determines eye and hair color and other traits inherited from our parents. In addition, genes ensure that we have two hands and can use them to do things, like play the piano."[25] Sometimes genetic defects, known as mutations, occur, which lead to the production of faulty proteins. This can cause cell malfunction, disease, and death. Many scientists believe that genetic mutation plays a role in the development of Alzheimer's disease and that more than one defective gene is

> **By the time someone has reached the age of 85, his or her chance of being stricken with [Alzheimer's] has risen to nearly 50 percent.**

involved. According to the NIA, researchers suspect that many forms of early-onset Alzheimer's are caused by genetic mutations on chromosomes 1, 14, or 21. An individual who inherits just one mutated gene from a parent is likely to develop early-onset Alzheimer's.

Unlike the early-onset type, late-onset Alzheimer's is not believed to be hereditary. So far, scientists have only identified one gene that could pose a risk for development of the disease, the apolipoprotein E gene, which is located on chromosome 19. The gene's function is to provide instructions for a lipoprotein that helps carry cholesterol and other fats through the bloodstream and delivers them to the proper locations in the body for processing and use. Researchers have learned that the apolipoprotein E gene is associated with plaques in the brain tissue of some people with Alzheimer's. This is not true in all cases, however, nor does everyone who has the gene develop the disease. Because so much is still unknown about the possible role of the gene in Alzheimer's disease, scientists continue to study it, along with other genetic risk factors. They suspect that there may be additional risk factors on chromosomes 9, 10, and 12, and they are closely studying those as well.

Alzheimer's and Other Diseases

Scientists have long known that people who suffer from certain chronic illnesses have a higher risk of developing Alzheimer's, and research continues to support this correlation. For instance, people with diabetes have been shown to have a 30 to 65 percent higher risk of developing Alzheimer's than those who are not diabetic. A characteristic of diabetes is that it causes blood glucose levels to be abnormally high, which can potentially have toxic effects on the brain and lead to the development of brain disease. In May 2008 researchers at the Salk Institute for Biological Studies published the results of a study on the molecular connection between diabetes and Alzheimer's. Diabetes was induced in young mice that had been genetically bred to acquire symptoms of Alzheimer's with old age.

> " Many scientists believe that genetic mutation plays a role in the development of Alzheimer's disease and that more than one defective gene is involved. "

The researchers found that blood vessels in the creatures' brains were damaged by the interaction of elevated blood glucose levels and the presence of beta amyloid. The damage occurred well before any signs of Alzheimer's, such as death of neurons or the presence of plaques, were detected. The researchers stated that even though all people have amyloid circulating in their bloodstreams, in diabetics there may be a toxicity between the protein and higher-than-normal levels of blood glucose.

Heart disease and high blood pressure are also believed to be risk factors for developing Alzheimer's. This was first discovered more than 20 years ago by a scientist named Larry Sparks, who was studying the brain tissue of people who had died. None of the victims had overt signs of dementia, but Sparks noticed that those who had plaques had one thing in common, as he explains: "I took the slides . . . and put them into two piles, those with heart disease and those without heart disease. And all the plaques and tangles showed up in the pile with heart disease."[26] In the years since his groundbreaking discovery, Sparks has directed many major research projects, one of which showed that high cholesterol is also linked to Alzheimer's. In one study, patients with high cholesterol and Alzheimer's were given a cholesterol-lowering medication known as Lipitor. Two-thirds of the participants derived some benefit from the drug; of those, many of their dementia symptoms either stabilized or improved.

> " Scientists have long known that people who suffer from certain chronic illnesses have a higher risk of developing Alzheimer's, and research continues to support this correlation. "

A study announced in June 2007 by researchers at the University Regional Hospital Center in Lille, France, showed that problems from heart disease can affect brain health. The research involved 891 French patients who were diagnosed with dementia, including Alzheimer's. At the start of the study, the research team gave the patients standard tests to measure their cognitive ability. Over the course of 36 months, some patients who suffered from cardiovascular disease were given cholesterol-lowering drugs or other medications, along with drugs aimed at temporarily curbing their dementia symptoms. Others in the group were not given the cardiovascular medications. When the study was concluded, the participants were again given cognitive tests. Those who were treated for vascular problems as well as dementia had no change in cognitive abilities, but the abilities of patients who did not receive vascular treatment severely deteriorated. Dr. Sam Gandy, the chairman of the Alzheimer's Association's National Medical and Scientific Advisory Council, says that the study represents "pretty exciting work" because it establishes that "treating vascular risk factors slows the progression of cognitive decline."[27]

Controversial Theories

Many scientists acknowledge that environmental factors likely play a role in the development of Alzheimer's disease, although exactly which factors are not known. According to the Mayo Clinic, researchers have studied, and continue to study, possible correlations between Alzheimer's and such hazards as smoking, exposure to pesticides and fertilizers, and even electromagnetic fields.

One of the most controversial theories is the role aluminum buildup in the body might play in development of Alzheimer's disease. Aluminum is a common element in Earth's crust and is found in numerous household products and personal care products, such as antiperspirant, as well as in antacids and many foods. The suspicion that aluminum could be linked to Alzheimer's arose during the 1960s, when scientists reportedly found that the injection of aluminum compounds into rabbits caused tanglelike formations in the creatures' nerve cells. It was discovered, however, that the tangles differed in structure and composition from the type that are found in the brains of people with Alzheimer's disease. According to the Alzheimer's Society in the United Kingdom, claims have been made that the brain content of aluminum is increased in people with Alzheimer's, but studies that compared Alzheimer's brains and normal brains failed to find any difference in the amount of the compounds. Although research has failed to find any causal relationship between aluminum and Alzheimer's disease, this is not a closed issue. Scientists continue to explore whether there might be some sort of connection.

> " One of the most controversial theories is the role aluminum buildup in the body might play in development of Alzheimer's disease. "

Another controversial theory is that flu vaccinations are linked to the onset of Alzheimer's. This began with a South Carolina doctor named Hugh Fudenberg, who claimed that people who had 5 consecutive flu shots between 1970 and 1980 had a risk of getting Alzheimer's that was 10 times higher than those who had only one or 2 shots. The Alzheimer's Association says that there is no scientific evidence that this is true, and several studies have actually linked flu shots and other vaccinations to a *reduced* risk of Alzheimer's.

An issue that continues to be debated is whether amalgams, silver dental fillings that contain mercury, increase the risk of Alzheimer's disease. According to the Alzheimer's Association, this is another misguided theory for which there is no tangible evidence. Not all scientists agree, however. In a September 2006 testimony before the U.S. Food and Drug Administration (FDA), Boyd Haley spoke about the risks of mercury and its possible link to Alzheimer's. Haley, who heads the chemistry department at the University of Kentucky and is an expert on mercury toxicity, stated that amalgams release toxic mercury into the mouth; if the mercury gets into the brain, this can lead to the formation of plaques and tangles. He added that anyone whose mouth has a significant number of amalgams would be at higher risk for developing Alzheimer's. One person who agrees with Haley's theory is Terry Pratchett, who believes that the old fillings in his teeth caused his disease, as he explains:

> I've got lots of fans in all parts of the world who, despite reading my books, have got fairly high up in the medical profession, and what I have been told is that a mouth that chews and crunches and fills with acid and then reacts with the mercury in your teeth is bound to have some impact. There's no medical evidence that the mercury amalgam in the fillings . . . causes Alzheimer's, but . . . I have had nearly all my metal fillings removed and replaced with those lovely white ones. I took advice from lots of people who I'm not going to name.[28]

Much Is Still Unknown

What causes Alzheimer's? Obviously it is a disease that primarily preys on the elderly, but why do some people get it while others do not? Research has shown connections between Alzheimer's and mutated genes, yet no studies have conclusively revealed exactly which genes contribute to the disease or why. There are also strong links between Alzheimer's and certain chronic illnesses, but that, too, raises as many questions as answers. The result of research continues to be promising, however, and more pieces of the Alzheimer's puzzle are falling into place. Perhaps in time the puzzle will be complete, and discovery of the cause will mean the beginning of the end for this devastating disease.

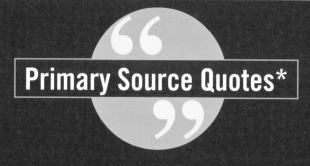

Primary Source Quotes*

What Causes Alzheimer's Disease?

66 The only way to confirm that someone has Alzheimer's disease . . . is by peering into their brains and seeing plaque, nestled between the twisted endings of affected nerve cells. Unfortunately, these markers can only be viewed during postmortem investigations. 99

—Nikhil Swaminathan, "Unraveling Alzheimer's Disease Plaques," *Scientific American*, February 6, 2008. www.sciam.com.

Swaminathan is a science writer from Brooklyn, New York.

66 Many people believe that you have to have the brain at autopsy before you can diagnose Alzheimer's, but that's not right. We do that for research, to confirm the diagnosis, but we can also identify the disease clinically with time and other tests. 99

—Eric Tangalos, "Diagnosing Alzheimer's: An Interview with a Mayo Clinic Specialist," MayoClinic.com, December 5, 2006. www.mayoclinic.com.

Tangalos is a primary care physician and geriatrician affiliated with the Alzheimer's Disease Research Center at the Mayo Clinic in Rochester, Minnesota.

Bracketed quotes indicate conflicting positions.

* Editor's Note: While the definition of a primary source can be narrowly or broadly defined, for the purposes of Compact Research, a primary source consists of: 1) results of original research presented by an organization or researcher; 2) eyewitness accounts of events, personal experience, or work experience; 3) first-person editorials offering pundits' opinions; 4) government officials presenting political plans and/or policies; 5) representatives of organizations presenting testimony or policy.

66 **Alzheimer's disease is devastating, and, despite great strides in recent years, still puzzling in its cause and mechanisms.** 99

—Vernon M. Ingram, "Alzheimer's Disease," *American Scientist*, July/August 2003. www.americanscientist.org.

Ingram is a professor of biology at the Massachusetts Institute of Technology.

66 **Scientists do not yet fully understand what causes Alzheimer's disease (AD). However, the more they learn about AD, the more they become aware of the important function genes play in the development of this devastating disease.** 99

—National Institute on Aging, "Alzheimer's Disease Genetics Fact Sheet," August 2004. www.nia.nih.gov.

The NIH supports and conducts research on aging processes, age-related diseases, and special problems and needs of the elderly.

66 **Only after you die and they pop open your head and inspect your deceased brain can they say for sure, sort of, if you had it.** 99

—Richard Taylor, *Alzheimer's from the Inside Out*. Baltimore: Health Professions, 2007.

Taylor is a retired psychologist who has Alzheimer's disease and acts as an advocate for improving Alzheimer's care.

66 **Even though we see these plaques and tangles in the postmortem brains of people with Alzheimer's, we don't know which come first. Scientists are unclear whether these structures cause the disease or whether they are a by-product of it. It's a chicken-or-the-egg problem.** 99

—Manny Alvarez, "Alzheimer's Disease: Betrayed by Your Brain," Fox News, February 21, 2007. www.foxnews.com.

Alvarez is managing editor of health news at Fox News as well as chairman of the Department of Obstetrics and Gynecology and Reproductive Science at Hackensack University Medical Center in New Jersey.

> 66 Dementia occurs in people with Alzheimer's disease because healthy brain tissue degenerates, causing a steady decline in memory and mental abilities. 99

—Mayo Clinic Staff, "Alzheimer's Disease," January 12, 2007. www.mayoclinic.com.

The Mayo Clinic is a world-renown medical facility that is dedicated to the diagnosis and treatment of virtually every type of illness.

> 66 Particular dietary habits, professional occupations, or personality types do not seem to lead to the development of Alzheimer's disease. 99

—Cognitive Neurology and Alzheimer's Disease Center, Northwestern University, "Alzheimer's Disease," October 2, 2006. www.brain.northwestern.edu.

The Cognitive Neurology and Alzheimer's Disease Center is dedicated to brain research, including disseminating the research to people with brain diseases and training researchers and clinicians.

> 66 Alzheimer's disease may be caused by something within the body. It could be a slow virus, an imbalance of chemicals or a problem with the immune system. 99

—Alzheimer Society of Canada, "Alzheimer's Disease," October 2005. www.alzheimer.ca.

The Alzheimer Society of Canada is a leading nonprofit health organization working to improve the quality of life for Canadians who are affected by Alzheimer's disease and also to advance research toward its cause and cure.

> 66 'Genetic' does not mean cast in stone. In no way is having a relative with Alzheimer's disease—even a genetically identical twin—a guarantee that a person is going to get Alzheimer's disease. 99

—Margaret Gatz, quoted in Louise Chang, "Who Gets Alzheimer's? Genes Hold Key," WebMD *Health*, February 6, 2006. www.medscape.com.

Gatz is a psychologist and researcher at the University of Southern California.

66 Many people with early-onset Alzheimer's have a parent or grandparent who also developed Alzheimer's at a younger age. A significant proportion of early-onset Alzheimer's is linked to three genes. 99

—Glenn Smith, "Early Onset Alzheimer's: When Symptoms Begin Before 65," Mayo Clinic, March 7, 2007. www.mayoclinic.com.

Smith is a board-certified clinical neuropsychologist who specializes in Alzheimer's disease.

66 It's reasonable to suppose that anything that is bad for your heart is bad for your brain, so it is no great surprise that secondhand smoke could be responsible for development of carotid artery disease and dementias of all kinds. 99

—Bill Thies, quoted in *Healthcare in the News*, "Secondhand Smoke Linked to Dementia," Reading Hospital and Medical Center, May 2, 2007. www.readinghospital.org.

Thies is the Alzheimer's Association's vice president for medical and scientific affairs.

What Causes Alzheimer's Disease?

- The likelihood of developing Alzheimer's disease doubles about every 5 years after age 65, and people over the age of 85 have almost a **50 percent** chance of developing Alzheimer's.

- Scientists have identified **one gene** that increases the risk of Alzheimer's, but it does not guarantee that someone will develop the disease.

- More than one **gene mutation** can cause Alzheimer's disease, and scientists believe that genes on multiple chromosomes are involved.

- In June 2007 researchers announced that the **death of brain cells due to head injury** could increase the risk of developing Alzheimer's disease.

- Research has shown that people with **heart disease, diabetes**, or **high blood pressure** are at greater risk of developing Alzheimer's.

- Researchers announced in March 2008 that a person's risk of developing Alzheimer's **doubles** if both parents have the disease.

- A study released in April 2008 showed that a **pattern of depression**, even decades earlier, can increase the risk for developing Alzheimer's.

- A 2008 study published in the medical journal *Neurology* stated that people who were overweight **with excessive belly fat** were at higher risk for developing Alzheimer's.

A Complex Illness

Scientists have been studying Alzheimer's for many years and they have learned a great deal about the disease. However, its exact cause still remains a mystery. It is believed to be caused by a variety of different factors working together.

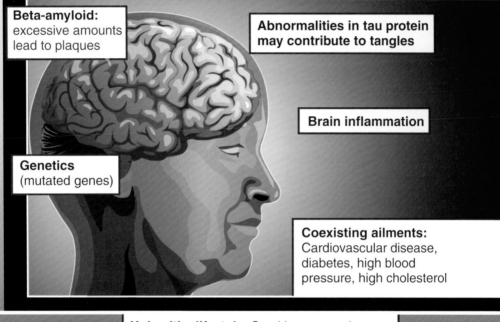

Beta-amyloid: excessive amounts lead to plaques

Abnormalities in tau protein may contribute to tangles

Brain inflammation

Genetics (mutated genes)

Coexisting ailments: Cardiovascular disease, diabetes, high blood pressure, high cholesterol

Unhealthy lifestyle: Smoking; excessive use of alcohol; lack of exercise, social stimulation, and mentally challenging activities

Source: National Institute on Aging, "Alzheimer's Disease: Unraveling the Mystery," December 2003. www.nia.nih.gov.

- Research has shown that over time damage from a type of molecule called a **free radical** can build up in neurons, leading to a loss in brain function.

- Researchers from the Netherlands found that the level of risk for developing Alzheimer's is **50 percent higher for smokers** than for non-smokers.

Age Is the Number-One Risk Factor

Scientists are aggressively pursuing research that will help them better understand the causes of Alzheimer's. Sometimes they disagree about theories, such as how much of a role plaques and tangles play, and whether they cause the disease or are a by-product of it. One thing scientists agree on, however, is that age, by far, is the greatest risk factor for someone to develop Alzheimer's. This graph shows that Alzheimer's cases increase with age.

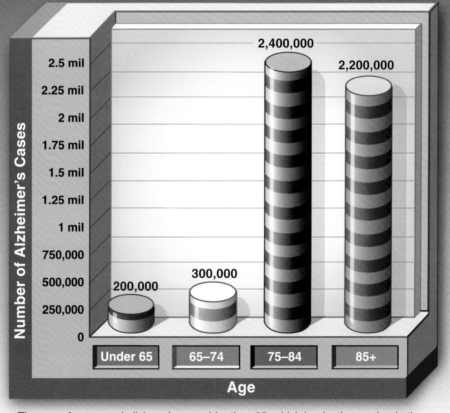

There are fewer people living who are older than 85, which is why the number in the 75–84 age bracket is higher than the 85+ bracket. Nearly 50 percent of Americans 85 years old and higher have Alzheimer's disease.

Source: Alzheimer's Association, "Media Fact Sheet—Greater San Francisco Bay Area," 2007. www.alz.org.

- In April 2008 researchers from the University of North Dakota announced that **caffeine in coffee** could lower the risk of dementia by blocking the damage caused by cholesterol.

Coexisting Medical Conditions

Scientists have learned that most people with Alzheimer's and other types of dementia have one or more other serious illnesses. This shows some of the medical conditions that are commonly associated with Alzheimer's disease.

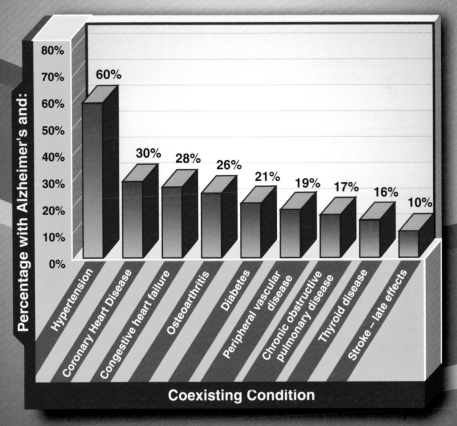

Source: Alzheimer's Association, "2008 Alzheimer's Disease Facts and Figures," August 2008. www.alz.org.

- In 2006 Columbia University researchers reported that people who followed a Mediterranean diet (large amounts of fruits, vegetables, beans, grains, and nuts) had a **40 to 65 percent lower risk** of developing Alzheimer's than people who did not follow the diet.

Who Suffers from Alzheimer's Disease?

Thomas DeBaggio was 57 years old when he was diagnosed with Alzheimer's disease in 1999. The owner of a thriving herb farm in northern Virginia, DeBaggio had become concerned when he could no longer remember the names of many of his plants. He also found that he "could not remember things that the year before had been brightly colored and detailed." Because of his relatively young age, he assumed that his newfound forgetfulness was caused by the stress of owning and operating his farm—yet deep inside his mind, he believed that something else was wrong. After telling his physician of his concerns, DeBaggio was referred for blood work and testing. When a neuropsychological evaluation diagnosed early-onset Alzheimer's and deemed his condition to be "severely impaired," he was devastated, as he explains: "At first I viewed the diagnosis as a death sentence. Tears welled up in my eyes uncontrollably; spasms of depression grabbed me by the throat. I was nearer to death than I anticipated." Then, a few days later, DeBaggio vowed to turn the horrible news into something positive by writing a book about it. "After forty years of pussyfooting with words," he writes, "I finally had a story of hell to tell."[29]

How Prevalent Is Alzheimer's Disease?

In its 2008 *Facts and Figures* report, the Alzheimer's Association presents sobering statistics. One startling fact is that every 71 seconds someone in America develops Alzheimer's. As of 2008, an estimated 5.2 million people in the United States suffered from the disease, including 2.4 million women and 1 million men over the age of 71. Yet far from being unique to the United States, Alzheimer's is a worldwide epidemic, affecting an estimated 26 million people throughout the world. The greatest number of Alzheimer's sufferers live in developing nations. Forty-eight percent of the world's Alzheimer's cases are currently found in Asian countries, for example, with the highest prevalence in India and China. Indeed, this disease has grown into a global health crisis that shows no signs of slowing down.

Because people throughout the world have a longer life expectancy than in the past, and since Alzheimer's is far more common among the elderly, the incidence of the disease is expected to soar in the future. In 2007 researchers from the Johns Hopkins Bloomberg School of Public Health released a study predicting that the worldwide prevalence of Alzheimer's would grow to more than 106 million by 2050. "We face a looming global epidemic of Alzheimer's disease

> " Because people throughout the world have a longer life expectancy than in the past, and since Alzheimer's is far more common among the elderly, the incidence of the disease is expected to skyrocket in the future. "

as the world's population ages," explains Ron Brookmeyer, the study's lead author. "By 2050, 1 in 85 persons worldwide will have Alzheimer's disease. However, if we can make even modest advances in preventing Alzheimer's disease or delay its progression, we could have a huge global public health impact."[30] Brookmeyer and his research team say that the largest increase in prevalence will occur in Asian countries. The number of Alzheimer's cases in Asia is expected to grow from 12.65 million in 2006 to nearly 63 million in 2050.

Are Racial Minorities at Greater Risk?

During the winter of 2008 Rutgers University released a publication titled "The Color of Risk," which focused on the disparity between Alzheimer's disease in Caucasians versus racial minorities. As author Daniel Pendick writes:

> The math couldn't be simpler—or crueler. African-Americans make up just 12 percent of the U.S. population, yet they are twice as likely as whites to develop Alzheimer's disease and 40 percent less likely to be properly diagnosed and treated. So when the long-forecasted 'Alzheimer's bomb' goes off in the aging American population, the faces will be disproportionately African.[31]

Many other researchers agree, estimating that the prevalence of Alzheimer's among black Americans is exponentially greater than it is among whites and could be as much as 100 percent higher. Other minority groups, such as Hispanics, are also at heightened risk when compared with society at large.

According to the Alzheimer's Association, though, while it is true that minorities are more likely than Caucasians to develop Alzheimer's, this can be explained by factors other than race. For example, it is widely known that cardiovascular disease, high cholesterol levels, high blood pressure, obesity, and diabetes are all factors that can increase someone's risk for Alzheimer's. Because minorities suffer from these ailments far more often than Caucasians, this could explain why they are so much more likely to have the disease. The organization explains: "Most analyses that have combined age, gender, . . . race, and other factors show that African-Americans do not have a statistically significant increased risk of dementia or that their increased risk in comparison with Caucasians is greatly reduced once these factors are taken into account."[32]

Another factor could be pertinent in explaining why black people are more likely to develop Alzheimer's than whites: education. One study of African Americans that was published in the journal *Archives of Neurology* showed that having fewer years of education was associated with a higher likelihood of having Alzheimer's and other dementias. One theory is that the brains of people with higher education may be better able to cope with the effects of the disease. The researchers stated that quality of education and socioeconomic factors that hinder access to education are probably more relevant than race in explaining why African Americans are more likely than Caucasians to develop Alzheimer's.

The Connection Between Alzheimer's and Down Syndrome

Down syndrome is a chromosomal disorder, with people afflicted by it having 47 chromosomes rather than the usual 46. Although no one knows why this occurs, researchers believe that those with Down syndrome have extra genetic material in chromosome 21. During the early twentieth century, babies who were born with Down syndrome died at a young age, often before they reached 10 years old. As treatments have improved over the years, the life expectancy for those with Down syndrome has markedly risen to about 56 years old. This is a mixed blessing, however, as people with the chromosomal disorder develop Alzheimer's disease at a much higher rate

> **One study of African Americans that was published in the journal *Archives of Neurology* showed that having fewer years of education was associated with a higher likelihood of having Alzheimer's and other dementias.**

than those who do not have the disorder. Researchers say that most, or even all, people with Down syndrome who live beyond a certain age will eventually develop Alzheimer's. According to Huntington Potter of the Byrd Alzheimer's Center and Research Institute in Tampa, Florida, "Every Down's syndrome individual who has three copies of chromosome 21 in every cell of their body develops Alzheimer's disease by the time they're 30 or 40."[33] The reason for this is mysterious to scientists, although research has spawned some theories.

Studies performed during the 1970s and 1980s showed that abnormalities seen in the brains of people with Alzheimer's also existed in the brains of those with Down syndrome. In one particular study, researchers examined 100 Down syndrome patients who had died and found that their brains were filled with plaques. Potter says that the gene that causes the excess amyloid proteins to build up in brains diseased by Alzheimer's is also contained on chromosome 21, the same chromosome that is triplicated in people with Down syndrome. He explains the significance: "Therefore, if you have three copies of the chromosome instead of only two, you'll have more of this bad protein and more accumulation and more damage."[34]

> **Researchers say that most, or even all, people with Down syndrome who live beyond a certain age will eventually develop Alzheimer's.**

Another researcher who studies the connection between Down syndrome and Alzheimer's disease is Colin Davidson, a geneticist at Stanford University. Davidson says that in both the brains of people with Alzheimer's and Down syndrome, the APP gene (part of chromosome 21) becomes mutated, which leads to the formation of plaques. He refers to research with laboratory mice that were bred to have the equivalent of Down syndrome. The study showed that the animals had increased levels of APP, and the way their brains were diseased resembled someone with Alzheimer's. "Of course, none of this is a smoking gun," Davidson says:

> While it is likely that people with Down syndrome have increased levels of the APP gene, this has yet to be proven. In addition, it is known that an extra APP gene is not enough to get Alzheimer's—there are more genes on chromosome 21 and other chromosomes involved.

So, while we know the genes responsible for Down syndrome, scientists are still trying to understand all the genes implicated in Alzheimer's disease.[35]

Children with Alzheimer's?

Although Alzheimer's is a disease that primarily afflicts the elderly, the early-onset type may affect people who are as young as in their thirties or forties. But a genetic disorder known as Niemann-Pick Type C strikes children—and those who are born with it develop dementia that is nearly identical to that of Alzheimer's. In children who are afflicted with Niemann-Pick, which is often referred to as Children's Alzheimer's, harmful amounts of fatty substances build up in the liver, spleen, bone marrow, and brain, causing much the same damage as plaques and tangles in the brain of someone with Alzheimer's. The disorder is extremely rare, affecting about 500 children worldwide each year. There is no cure, and most of those stricken with it do not live past the age of 20.

Leah Garfitt is a seven-year-old girl from the United Kingdom who was diagnosed with Niemann-Pick when she was a year old. The first symptoms her mother noticed were that the little girl's eyesight was failing, she stumbled often, and forgot even the simplest words she had previously learned. After she was diagnosed, doctors told Leah's mother that the child's condition would continue to deteriorate, she would lose her sight and hearing, would lose muscle tone that would render her unable to walk or swallow, and full-blown dementia would set in before she reached her teenage years. "She already has all the symptoms of senile dementia," her mother said in January 2008. "It is a really terrible disease."[36]

> As much as [Alzheimer's patients] suffer, by the time they have reached the advanced stages of their disease, their families are likely to suffer more than they do.

Another child from the United Kingdom who suffers from Niemann-Pick is two-year-old Taylor Smith, who was diagnosed when he was 14 months old. As of May 2008 Taylor had not developed any obvious symptoms of the disease, but his mother, Stephanie O'Hara, feels as though she is "living with a timebomb" because she realizes that it is only a matter of time before signs of dementia start to appear. "It's heartbreaking to see Taylor learning all these new skills but knowing they will be taken away from him as the disease sets in," she says. "But we are just taking each day as it comes and trying to make Taylor's life the best it can be."[37]

"I Can Hardly Stand to Think About It"

When people are diagnosed with Alzheimer's disease, it is a crushing blow. They wonder how long it will be before they can no longer remember anything that they once knew, or how much time will pass before their minds are completely gone. Yet as much as they suffer, by the time they have reached the advanced stages of their disease, their families are likely to suffer more than they do. The Alzheimer's patient often retreats to a more peaceful place, where he or she is removed from much of the agony caused by the disease. Patti Davis, the daughter of former president Ronald Reagan, shares her experience with this: "By the time it was clear that my father really wasn't sure who I was . . . he had drifted into a softer, more comfortable realm."[38] Families, however, often do not find peace during this time. It is they who must watch someone they love slip further and further away from them until every spark of life seems to have been snuffed out. It is they who must cope with knowing that their loved one no longer knows them, and will never know them again. It is they who must accept the fact that Alzheimer's will inevitably claim the life of someone they have loved for many years.

Brenda van Dyck experienced this when her father was stricken with Alzheimer's disease. It started in the usual way: He began forgetting things and easily became confused. When the symptoms grew worse, his memory continued to fail, and he often became lost, van Dyck knew that this was much more than just normal aging. Soon afterward her father was diagnosed with Alzheimer's, and she shares what it is like to witness his deterioration: "The disease has already taken so much of him away; it's like looking at a jigsaw puzzle; you can make out the whole picture with just a few pieces missing, but when more and more pieces get lost, it's hard to tell what the picture is." Van Dyck copes with her father's steady decline by clinging to memories of him, but that, too, is painful for her, as she explains: "He was so capable. It seemed he could do anything. He used to harvest a bevy of vegetables from his garden all summer long, change the oil in the car, bake hearty wheat bread, build things around the house. I miss that man. So many puzzle pieces are gone now that the picture looks entirely different. I can hardly stand to think about it."[39]

Will the Suffering End?

Alzheimer's disease strikes people all over the world. It is most common in the elderly, but younger people may be afflicted by it as well. In extremely rare cases, children can even be born with a genetic disorder that, like Alzheimer's, leads to dementia and death. Families suffer as they watch their loved ones slip away, one memory at a time. Researchers predict that with the fast-growing aging population, the number of people who suffer from Alzheimer's will quadruple by the year 2050. Their hope is that they can stop this tragic disease long before then, and they continue to work aggressively to make that happen.

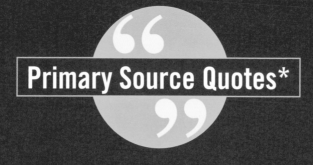

Primary Source Quotes*

Who Suffers from Alzheimer's Disease?

66 Every 71 seconds, someone in America develops Alzheimer's disease. By mid-century, someone will develop Alzheimer's every 33 seconds. 99

—Alzheimer's Association, "2008 Alzheimer's Disease Facts and Figures," August 2008. www.alz.org.

The Alzheimer's Association is a health organization that seeks to eliminate Alzheimer's disease through research as well as provide and enhance care and support for those who have the disease.

66 If the onset of Alzheimer's could be delayed by five years, the projected population that is expected to suffer from the disease could be cut in half. 99

—Daniel Perry and Carol Schutz, "Friends of the National Institute on Aging Testimony on FY 2008 National Institutes of Health Appropriations," March 30, 2007. www.agingresearch.org.

Perry is chair of the Alliance for Aging Research, and Schutz is cochair of the Gerontological Society of America.

* Editor's Note: While the definition of a primary source can be narrowly or broadly defined, for the purposes of Compact Research, a primary source consists of: 1) results of original research presented by an organization or researcher; 2) eyewitness accounts of events, personal experience, or work experience; 3) first-person editorials offering pundits' opinions; 4) government officials presenting political plans and/or policies; 5) representatives of organizations presenting testimony or policy.

**66 At least 200,000 under age 65—or 5 percent to 10 per-
cent of Alzheimer's victims—suffer from the disease.
Active, athletic parents with young children and high-
profile jobs are finding they have the disease. 99**

—Claude Solnik, "Alzheimer's Invisible Victims," *Long Island (NY) Business News*, May 2, 2008.

Solnik is a staff writer for *Long Island Business News*.

....

**66 Alzheimer's cases are due to double in the next gener-
ation. It is a disease that leaves you a shell of yourself.
The buoyantly healthy baby boomers are staying alive
long enough to drop right into its lair. 99**

—Terry Pratchett, "Boomers' Little Secret," *Newsweek International*, April 21, 2008. www.newsweek.com.

Pratchett is a science-fiction writer from the United Kingdom who was diagnosed
with a rare form of early-onset Alzheimer's disease at the age of 59.

....

**66 Known by many as 'the long goodbye,' Alzheimer's dis-
ease is increasing at an alarming rate in the United
States. 99**

—Carrie Hill, "What Is Alzheimer's?" About.com, May 7, 2008. http://alzheimers.about.com.

Hill is a writer who was formerly the regional director of the Alzheimer's Association in southern Utah.

....

**66 There are currently over 4,000,000 families dealing
with Alzheimer's in the U.S. alone. By 2010, that number is projected to be over 10,000,000. 99**

—Alzheimer's Research Foundation, "Helpful Hints: What's This All About?" www.alzheimers-research.org.

The Alzheimer's Research Foundation investigates Alzheimer's causes, treatments, and cures, and supports services for caregivers and patients' families.

....

❝Alzheimer's disease, one of the most frightening memory-robbing disorders, hampers the lives of some 4 to 5 million older Americans.❞

—Carol Barnes, "Testimony on Behalf of the Society for Neuroscience," March 22, 2005. www.sfn.org.

Barnes is the former president of the Society for Neuroscience.

❝Everyone knows Alzheimer's is a looming public health epidemic because of the aging of the population.❞

—Peter Snyder, quoted in PR Newswire, "Landmark Alzheimer's Report Urges Radical Changes to Paradigm of Therapy Development for Alzheimer's Disease and Dementias to Focus on Prevention," May 15, 2008. www.prnewswire.com.

Snyder is a professor in the Department of Psychology at the University of Connecticut.

❝If we all live to be a 120 probably most of us would have Alzheimer's disease and people who live to be 100 about 6 out of 10 have got clear symptoms of Alzheimer's disease, where at the age of 60/65 it's only about 1 in 100.❞

—David Ames, "Alzheimer's, Testosterone, and the Ageing Brain," *Health Report*, May 21, 2007. www.abc.net.au.

Ames is the principal investigator of the Australian Imaging Biomarkers and Lifestyle Study in Melbourne, Australia.

❝It is generally recognized that the prevalence of Alzheimer's disease is higher in women, but whether incidence is increased in women remains a controversial issue.❞

—Anil Nair, "Top 5 Dementia Myths Debunked," *HealthTalk*, June 13, 2007. www.bu.edu.

Nair is an assistant professor of neurology at Boston University School of Medicine.

❝Alzheimer's is going to swamp the health care system.❞

—John C. Morris, quoted in Denise Grady, "Link Between Alzheimer's and Diabetes Deepens," *New York Times*, July 17, 2006. www.nytimes.com.

Morris is a neurology professor at Washington University in St. Louis and an adviser to the Alzheimer's Association.

❝It is frightening to lose control of your body in any way. It is especially tragic when the body's central control system, the brain, is the target of an angry destructive process that science has been unable to tame or reclaim.❞

—Thomas DeBaggio, *Losing My Mind: An Intimate Look at Life with Alzheimer's*. New York: Free Press, 2002.

DeBaggio, an artist and the owner of an herb farm in northern Virginia, was diagnosed with Alzheimer's disease when he was 57 years old.

Facts and Illustrations

Who Suffers from Alzheimer's Disease?

- The Alzheimer's Association states that one in 8 persons aged 65 and older (**13 percent**) suffers from Alzheimer's disease.

- In people aged 90 and older, Alzheimer's disease accounts for **80 percent** of all dementias, compared to **47 percent** for people aged 71 through 79.

- An estimated **67 percent** of people with Alzheimer's live in developing countries.

- According to the Alzheimer's Association, an estimated **10 million baby boomers** (people living in the United States who were born between 1946 and 1964) will develop Alzheimer's disease in their lifetime.

- A 2007 report in the journal *Neuroepidemiology* showed that **16 percent** of women and **11 percent** of men over the age of 71 have some form of dementia.

- The Alzheimer's Association states that more women have Alzheimer's and other dementias than men because **women live longer**.

- According to studies presented in 2004 at the Ninth International Conference on Alzheimer's Disease and Related Disorders, Alzheimer's disease symptoms begin an average of almost seven years earlier in **U.S. Latinos** than they do in Caucasians.

The Aging American Population

Because of advances in technology and medical care, people are living longer now than ever before. Since the early twentieth century the number of older adults has steadily increased and experts predict that the numbers will rise dramatically in the future. One reason for this projected increase is that the baby boomers (those born between 1946 and 1964) will begin turning 65 in 2011. This graph shows the actual and projected growth of the American population aged 65 and older. As the population ages, the number of people with Alzheimer's is expected to soar.

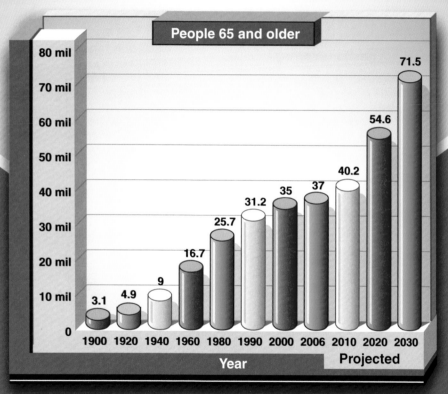

People 65 and older

Year	People 65 and older (mil)
1900	3.1
1920	4.9
1940	9
1960	16.7
1980	25.7
1990	31.2
2000	35
2006	37
2010	40.2
2020	54.6
2030	71.5

Projected

Sources: Federal Interagency Forum on Aging-Related Statistics, "Older Americans 2008." www.aoa.gov; National Institute on Aging, "Alzheimer's Disease: Unraveling the Mystery," December 2003.

- According to the National Down Syndrome Society, the risk of developing Alzheimer's disease is **three to five times** greater in people with **Down syndrome** than it is in the general population.

Women More Likely to Suffer from Alzheimer's Disease

More women than men have Alzheimer's, although this may be because women typically live longer. Whatever the reason, the Alzheimer's Association estimates that women have a higher lifetime risk of being stricken with Alzheimer's and other dementias if they live to be at least 55 years old.

Percentage of women and men who will develop some form of dementia in their lifetime if they live to be at least 55

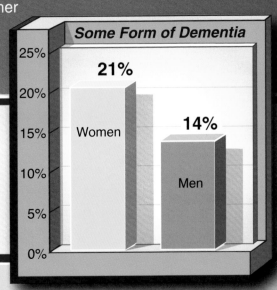

Some Form of Dementia

- Women: 21%
- Men: 14%

Percentage of women and men who will develop Alzheimer's disease in their lifetime if they live to be at least 55

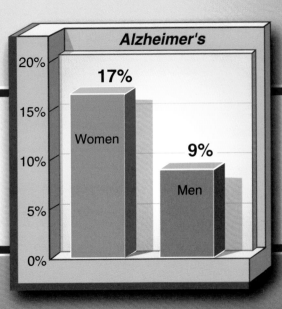

Alzheimer's

- Women: 17%
- Men: 9%

Source: Alzheimer's Association, "2008 Alzheimer's Disease Facts and Figures," August 2008. www.alz.org.

Americans Fear Alzheimer's

A January 2006 survey by Harris Interactive showed that Alzheimer's is the second most feared illness in America, behind cancer. The survey involved 1,008 adults (503 men and 505 women) aged 18 or older who were given a list of diseases and asked to state which they feared the most. This graph shows how they responded.

20 percent
Alzheimer's Disease

14 percent
Heart Disease

38 percent
Cancer

13 percent
Stroke

9 percent
Diabetes

6 percent
Other

Source: Metlife, "Metlife Foundation Alzheimer's Survey: What America Thinks," May 11, 2006. www.metlife.com.

- Research has shown that nearly all Down syndrome patients have the brain changes associated with Alzheimer's disease by the time they reach the age of **40**.

- According to the Alzheimer's Assocation, in 2004 deaths rates for people with Alzheimer's disease varied by ethnicity. Caucasian females had the highest rates (**24.7 deaths** per 100,000 people), African American females were next (**19.9 deaths** per 100,000), and Hispanic males had the lowest death rates (**10.8 deaths** per 100,000).

Leading Causes of Death

Alzheimer's disease is among the top 10 leading causes of death for people of all ages, and is the fifth cause of death for those who are 65 and older. This graph shows how some other causes of death have decreased since 2000, while in the same period Alzheimer's-related deaths have soared.

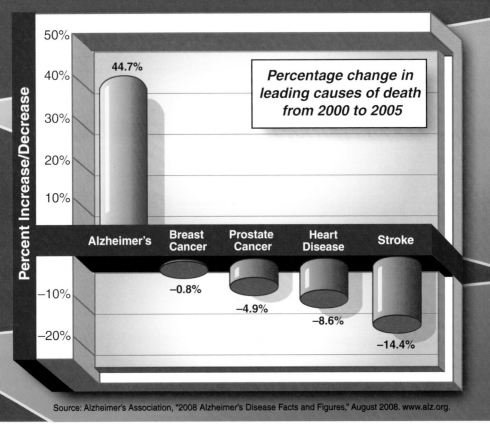

Percentage change in leading causes of death from 2000 to 2005

44.7% — Alzheimer's
−0.8% — Breast Cancer
−4.9% — Prostate Cancer
−8.6% — Heart Disease
−14.4% — Stroke

Source: Alzheimer's Association, "2008 Alzheimer's Disease Facts and Figures," August 2008. www.alz.org.

- According to the Centers for Disease Control and Prevention, of all the U.S. states, Washington has the highest number of deaths due to Alzheimer's disease at **36.1** per 100,000, followed by North Dakota at **33.5**, and Maine at **32.4**.

Will Research Prevent or Cure Alzheimer's Disease?

> **A cure for Alzheimer's disease remains a holy grail for a growing number of scientists and medical researchers around the globe.**
>
> —Fisher Center for Alzheimer's Research Foundation, "In Search of an Alzheimer's Cure."

> **My prayer is that a cure will be found so that no one else will have to endure being robbed of themselves, and no other families will be deprived of their loved ones because of Alzheimer's disease.**
>
> —Christina Fuller, "The Wedding Crasher."

For the millions of people who suffer from Alzheimer's, as well as their families, and all the older adults who live in fear of the disease, research cannot possibly progress fast enough. So much has been learned throughout the years, but many questions still remain unanswered. Scientists all over the world know that Alzheimer's is expected to reach epidemic proportions in the not-so-distant future. That is why they are aggressively searching for its cause and trying to develop drugs that will treat it, prevent its onset, and eventually eradicate it altogether. Maria Torroella Carney, who is commissioner of health in Nassau County, New York, shares her views:

More research is needed to learn how to prevent the development, slow the progression and manage the symptoms of Alzheimer's Disease. We need to more clearly understand why and how Alzheimer's Disease occurs and who is at greatest risk. The ability to accurately identify those at risk and diagnose the disease early is imperative so treatments can be initiated as early as possible to reduce the severity of the disease. . . . The time is now.[40]

Improved Diagnostic Tools

Scientists often say that the earlier Alzheimer's disease is discovered, before plaques and tangles have taken over the brain, the more effective treatments will be. Dr. Sam Gandy explains: "The most intensive area of Alzheimer's research right now is to determine how to slow the progression of it years or even decades before the plaques start to cause symptoms."[41] That will only be possible, however, if researchers find ways to detect Alzheimer's disease as early as possible. Thus, they continue to search for more sophisticated diagnostic tools.

A discovery made in 2002, and research that followed it, led to the development of a tool that could eventually be used to diagnose Alzheimer's before it has caused extensive damage to the brain. By examining the eyes of patients who had died of Alzheimer's, Lee Goldstein, a psychiatrist at Brigham and Women's Hospital in Boston, found that the same plaques that had ravaged the brain were visible around the rim of the lens of the eyes. Goldstein went on to develop a special two-part eye test: fluorescent eye drops that will bind to the plaques and a high-tech light-scattering laser device that can be used to examine a patient's eyeball. Because there are eye drops involved, the test must be approved by the FDA before it can be used in human clinical trials. Still, scientists are excited about the development because, as Goldstein explains, "if we can get treatments early . . . we can slow the disease to the point where we've effectively cured it."[42]

> **Scientists all over the world know that Alzheimer's is expected to reach epidemic proportions in the not-so-distant future.**

In March 2008 a team of researchers in Bedford, Massachusetts, announced that it had developed a way to examine brain tissue with near-infrared light. This technology has the ability to safely penetrate the skull while passing harmlessly through the brain. Although some of the light scatters, *how* it scatters can tell researchers about conditions in the brain. In a paper published in the journal *Optics Letters*, the team describes how it used near-infrared light to study tissue samples that were taken from different autopsies. Upon examination researchers were able to correctly identify which samples came from people who had Alzheimer's because the optical technology allowed them to detect the presence of plaques. The next step will be testing the technique for its effectiveness at diagnosing Alzheimer's disease in people who are alive.

> **Researchers at New York's Weill Cornell Medical College discovered a pattern of 23 proteins floating in spinal fluid that seemed to identify the presence of Alzheimer's disease.**

Another potential diagnostic tool was announced in December 2006. Researchers at New York's Weill Cornell Medical College discovered a pattern of 23 proteins floating in spinal fluid that seemed to identify the presence of Alzheimer's disease. Using a technology called proteomics, they examined 2,000 proteins found in the spinal fluid of 34 people who had died from Alzheimer's, and compared it to the spinal fluid of 34 people who had died of other causes. They discovered the 23 proteins that formed a "fingerprint" of the disease. Then they looked for that same protein pattern in the spinal fluid of 28 other people, and in 9 out of 10 cases, they were able to identify which people had Alzheimer's and which did not. The results of the study were promising, and it is hoped that it could possibly lead to scientists being able to detect Alzheimer's at an early stage by extracting spinal fluid from living patients.

"Rapid Widespread Effects"

In January 2008 an exciting discovery was announced by Edward L. Tobinick of California's Institute for Neurological Research. In a case report published in the *Journal of Neuroinflammation*, Tobinick discussed an experimental drug therapy that showed immense potential for treating Alzheimer's. It is his theory that the primary cause of the Alzheimer's disease is inflammation in the brain, which in turn adversely affects synapse transmission among neurons. In a pilot study conducted during 2006, he gave an 81-year-old male Alzheimer's patient injections of etanercept, which is usually used to treat inflammation and arthritis. Prior to the injection the man was given a variety of cognitive tests. Even though he was a retired physician who had years of medical education, he could not do simple mathematical calculations: When asked to add 29 plus 11, he answered 31. When asked to list all the animals he could in 60 seconds, he was only able to name dog and cat. He did not know which state he lived in or what year it was. After repeatedly being told the name of a physician, he had forgotten the name after 90 seconds. The man also failed at solving abstract concepts, such as how a train and a bicycle, a watch and a ruler, or music and painting were similar to each other.

> **Many scientists believe that the answer to an Alzheimer's cure lies with stem cells, the body's master cells from which all other cells are created.**

Remarkable changes were obvious just 10 minutes after he was given injections of etanercept. Tobinick writes that the man was "noticeably calmer, less frustrated, and more attentive. He was able to correctly identify the state as California, and he knew that the year was 2006. His responses to questioning seemed less effortful and more rapid, with less latency." Two hours after the treatment the man showed even more improvement. He identified that a train and a bicycle were similar because they were both used for transportation, and he said that a watch and a ruler were alike in that they both provided information. He said that painting was something that was done by hand, and music was heard with the ears. The man returned to the clinic a week later for further testing, and his cognitive skills were still much sharper than they had been before the treatment. In fact, his progress was obvious enough that his wife and son told Tobinick they had observed marked improvement throughout the week. During that examination, the man correctly identified the year, month, day of the week, the current season, and the state in which he lived. When asked to list all of the words that started with the letter F in 60 seconds, he listed 8 words, and also named 6 animals in 60 seconds. Based on this study, and others that showed similar results, Tobinick concluded that the use of etanercept with Alzheimer's patients "might have rapid widespread effects." He added that such research was "worthy of further investigation, and may lead to earlier therapeutic intervention which may have the potential to favorably affect the natural history of Alzheimer's disease."[43]

The Potential of Stem Cells

Many scientists believe that the answer to an Alzheimer's cure lies with stem cells, the body's master cells from which all other cells are created. Unlike regular cells that have specialized purposes, such as carrying oxygen through the blood or keeping the immune system strong, stem cells are pluripotent, meaning they have the ability to change into many other types of cells. Adult stem cells are found throughout the bodies of children and adults, everywhere from the spongy tissue inside bones (bone marrow) to the brain, heart, liver, lymph nodes, blood vessels, and skin. They are also found in umbilical cord blood and placenta. Embryonic stem cells come from embryos; specifically, four- to six-day-old embryos that are known as blastocysts. These are usually left over after parents undergo fertility treatments at clinics and donate their spare embryos for research.

Scientists are pursuing all kinds of stem cell research, but many are convinced that the greatest potential for Alzheimer's disease is with embryonic stem cells. In June 2005 Larry Goldstein gave testimony before the U.S. Senate Special Committee on Aging. Goldstein explained the urgency of Alzheimer's research and shared his thoughts about the crucial role stem cells play. He stated:

> I am here today to discuss how my research, and that of other scientists, is trying to take advantage of the enormous scientific and medical opportunity provided by human embryonic stem cells. I want to be cautious and

stress that scientific progress in the fight against diseases such as Alzheimer's is difficult and sometimes agonizingly slow—even when the best tools are available. . . . Nonetheless, I and many of my colleagues think that human embryonic stem cells potentially hold the key to major advances in the search for new understanding of, and new treatments for, these terrible diseases.[44]

The goal of stem cell research is for scientists to eventually repair the brains of people with Alzheimer's by inducing embryonic stem cells to become the types of brain cells that are damaged by the disease. This has already been accomplished in animals by researchers at the Harvard Medical School. After the brains of elderly and brain-damaged mice were implanted with stem cells, neurons began to heal, new neurons grew, and there was a significant improvement in the creatures' brain function. Researcher Evan Snyder explains: "It's not unreasonable to think that in humans the early implantation of stem cells—because of the partnerships they form with host cells—might forestall or even pre-empt degenerative diseases such as Parkinson's and Alzheimer's. Perhaps, attacks by such diseases could be made less ferocious and mild enough for patients to adapt."[45]

> " As promising as Alzheimer's research has been, and continues to be, many scientists are frustrated over what they see as inadequate federal funding compared with allocations for other diseases and disorders. "

Is Alzheimer's Research Underfunded?

As promising as Alzheimer's research has been, and continues to be, many scientists are frustrated over what they see as inadequate federal funding compared with allocations for other diseases and disorders. For instance, in 2005 (the last year for which mortality data are available) 17,011 people in the United States died of AIDS and 40,870 people died of breast cancer. In its fiscal year 2009 funding report, the NIH allocated an estimated $2.9 billion for HIV/AIDS research, and $703 million for breast cancer. Alzheimer's disease, which claimed the lives of 71,696 people in 2005—nearly double that of breast cancer and more than quadruple the number of AIDS deaths—was granted $644 million in NIH funding. This was also less than allocations given for cancer ($5.7 billion), infectious disease ($3 billion), substance abuse ($1.5 billion), digestive diseases ($1.2 billion), diabetes ($1 billion), and obesity ($658 million). Another consideration is that even though Alzheimer's cases grew from 4.5 million in 2002 to 5.4 million in 2008, federal funding increased only slightly. If Alzheimer's becomes the public health crisis that scientists predict it will, more adequate funding for research will be crucial.

John C. Morris, director of the Alzheimer's disease research center at Washington University in St. Louis, believes that there is tremendous potential to find treatments and cures for Alzheimer's disease. He cautions, however, that this will not happen if researchers are inhibited by low funding. He explains:

> One irony is that the past two decades of Alzheimer's research have brought us to the point where we now have multiple drugs and interventions with the potential to be truly effective in treating Alzheimer's, but just as we finally have reached this optimistic point, the federal funding to support Alzheimer research actually is declining! Hence, opportunities to thoroughly evaluate promising new agents and develop new lines of research are being squandered. Even more problematic, new investigators are discouraged by this dire funding climate and are leaving the field, making me very worried that we are losing the "next generation" of Alzheimer's researchers. Research must be supported so that we can conquer Alzheimer's before it overwhelms our health care system.[46]

Challenges and Hope

If the scourge of Alzheimer's is ever going to be eliminated, it will be because of progressive scientific research. An in-depth understanding of the causes, more precise diagnostic methods, and treatments that delay onset and alleviate symptoms are all crucial in the fight against this disease that haunts millions of people all over the world. Will the day come when Alzheimer's is as rare as polio, measles, or diphtheria, or as nonexistent as smallpox? Although that is not known for sure, scientists are certainly optimistic about it. They vow to keep fighting because any disease that robs people of their minds is tragic enough to merit every bit of effort and attention it receives.

Primary Source Quotes*

Will Research Prevent or Cure Alzheimer's Disease?

"I cannot over-emphasize the need for urgency. The families of people with Alzheimer's disease are impatient for new treatment options that can offer new hope to them and their loved ones. We must resolve, by our swift action, that the current generation of people with Alzheimer's will be the last generation that we lose to this miserable disease."

—Sandra Day O'Connor, "Statement of Sandra Day O'Connor," *The Future of Alzheimer's: Breakthroughs and Challenges*, U.S. Senate Special Committee on Aging, May 14, 2008. http://aging.senate.gov.

O'Connor is a retired associate justice of the U.S. Supreme Court whose husband is in the advanced stages of Alzheimer's disease.

"Our vision is a world without Alzheimer's disease."

—Alzheimer's Association, "2008 Alzheimer's Disease Facts and Figures," August 2008. www.alz.org.

The Alzheimer's Association is a health organization that seeks to eliminate Alzheimer's disease through research as well as to provide and enhance care and support for those who have the disease.

* Editor's Note: While the definition of a primary source can be narrowly or broadly defined, for the purposes of Compact Research, a primary source consists of: 1) results of original research presented by an organization or researcher; 2) eyewitness accounts of events, personal experience, or work experience; 3) first-person editorials offering pundits' opinions; 4) government officials presenting political plans and/or policies; 5) representatives of organizations presenting testimony or policy.

66 **Alzheimer's is a crisis that mounts by the day. We have let too many of these days slip by without bold, decisive action to deliver meaningful relief to the millions of Americans struggling with this terrible disease.** 99

—Newt Gingrich, "Statement of Newt Gingrich," *The Future of Alzheimer's: Breakthroughs and Challenges,* U.S. Senate Special Committee on Aging, May 14, 2008. http://aging.senate.gov.

Gingrich is the former Speaker of the U.S. House of Representatives.

66 **Scientific progress in the fight against diseases such as Alzheimer's is difficult and sometimes agonizingly slow—even when the best tools are available; importantly, guarantees are hard to come by.** 99

—Larry Goldstein, "Testimony of Larry Goldstein, Ph.D.," June 8, 2005. www.isscr.org.

Goldstein is a professor of cellular and molecular medicine at the University of California, San Diego, School of Medicine.

66 **Unfortunately funding for Alzheimer research has declined every year for the last four years. Good scientific ideas are not being researched, young scientists and their new ideas are not being funded and life-saving treatments are being delayed or potentially lost forever.** 99

—Chuck Jackson, "Statement of Chuck Jackson," *The Future of Alzheimer's: Breakthroughs and Challenges,* U.S. Senate Special Committee on Aging, May 14, 2008. http://aging.senate.gov.

Jackson is a man from Albany, Oregon, who has been diagnosed with early-onset Alzheimer's disease.

66 **We await, together with the rest of the world, for new drugs that may some day be able to treat the underlying cause of this insidious disease as well as other neurological diseases, not just the symptoms.** 99

—Andrew C. von Eschenbach, "Alzheimer's Disease: FDA's Role in New Product Development," testimony to the U.S. Senate, July 17, 2007. www.fda.gov.

Von Eschenbach is commissioner of food and drugs for the U.S. Food and Drug Administration.

66 Even if current research yields new drugs, there is not likely to be a miracle pill that will bring people back from deep dementia. For now, there is no choice but to cope with the disease. 99

—Denise Grady, "Finding Alzheimer's Before a Mind Fails," *New York Times*, December 26, 2007. www.nytimes.com.

Grady is an award-winning science journalist who writes for the *New York Times*.

66 Ten years ago, we had essentially no idea about the mechanism of Alzheimer's disease. Since then, the ability to look under the hood has revealed key causative mechanisms and it has led to an explosion of drug development. I believe that we will see drugs emerge that can prevent Alzheimer's before symptoms occur. 99

—Eric Lander, "Federal Research Funding Testimony," American Society for Cell Biology, 2008. www.ascb.org.

Lander is a professor of biology at the Massachusetts Institute of Technology (MIT) and the director of the Whitehead Institute/MIT Center for Genome Research.

66 A lot of research is currently being done on Alzheimer's —we're studying genetic links and looking at molecules that might be destroying healthy brain tissue— and we're hopeful that this science will ultimately lead to a cure. 99

—William J. Hall, "Dr. Hall on Living with Alzheimer's," *Revolution Health*, January 31, 2007. www.revolutionhealth.com.

Hall is director of the Center for Healthy Aging and a professor of medicine at the University of Rochester School of Medicine.

> **"Alzheimer's disease is a complicated illness, so many research approaches almost certainly will be needed before the disease is more completely understood. However, a great deal has been learned in the past two decades."**

John C. Morris, "Readers' Questions: Alzheimer's Disease," *New York Times*, December 26, 2007. http://science.blogs.nytimes.com.

Morris is director of the Alzheimer's disease research center at Washington University in St. Louis.

> **"Compared to even a decade ago, the field of neuroscience is moving at an extraordinary pace. We know, however, breakthroughs cannot come quickly enough for the millions of Americans touched by Alzheimer's disease."**

—Elias A. Zerhouni, "NIH Research on Alzheimer's Disease and Other Cognitive Disorders," to the Committee on Health, Education, Labor, and Pensions, Subcommittee on Retirement and Aging, U.S. Senate, July 17, 2007. www.hhs.gov.

Zerhouni is director of the National Institutes of Health.

> **"I really want people to understand the progress we've made in the last 20 years, and I want them to share in the excitement of it. We went from being totally in the dark about Alzheimer's to having a deep understanding at the molecular level of what's going wrong in the brain— enough so that we can now develop highly specialized drugs that go right to the root of the problem."**

—Rudolph Tanzi, "An Interview with Dr. Rudolph Tanzi," China Millennium Council, 2005. www.chinafrontier.com.

Tanzi is a professor of neurology at Harvard University Medical School whose primary specialty is Alzheimer's disease research.

Facts and Illustrations

Will Research Prevent or Cure Alzheimer's Disease?

- The direct and indirect costs of Alzheimer's and other dementias total more than **$148 billion** per year; by 2025, the number is predicted to soar to **$400 billion**.

- Medicare currently spends nearly **three times** as much for people with Alzheimer's and other dementias than it does for average Medicare beneficiaries.

- Medicare costs are projected to double from $91 billion in 2005 to more than **$189 billion** by 2015, which, according to the Alzheimer's Association, is more than the current gross national product of **86 percent** of the world's countries.

- Researchers announced in January 2008 the development of a therapeutic molecule that could potentially prevent the formation of plaque in the brain; human clinical trials showed marked improvement in Alzheimer's patients within **minutes of administration**.

- Researchers at the Wellcome Trust Centre for Neuroimaging in London announced in February 2008 that they could diagnose Alzheimer's using MRI brain scans with **accuracy as high at 96 percent**.

The Promise of Stem Cells

Scientists throughout the world believe that stem cells hold the potential for innumerable treatments and cures for diseases, one of which is Alzheimer's. Stem cells are the master cells of the body, and have the ability to change into other cell types. In December 2007 researchers found that they could generate stem cells from common adult skin cells —a breakthrough discovery, as it could mean that stem cells derived from neurons of people with Alzheimer's could potentially be coaxed into growing new, healthy neurons in laboratory petri dishes. This illustration shows how such a process might work.

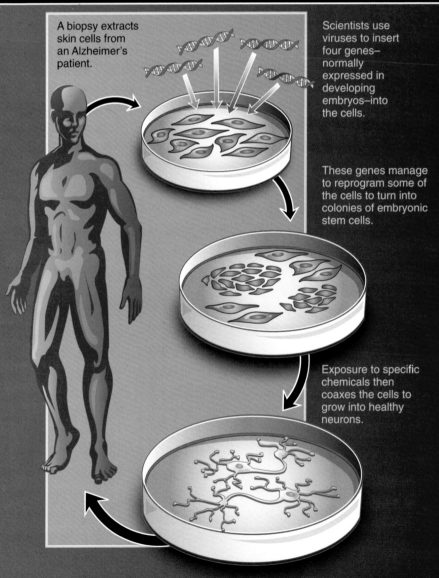

A biopsy extracts skin cells from an Alzheimer's patient.

Scientists use viruses to insert four genes— normally expressed in developing embryos—into the cells.

These genes manage to reprogram some of the cells to turn into colonies of embryonic stem cells.

Exposure to specific chemicals then coaxes the cells to grow into healthy neurons.

Source: *Technology Review*, "Customized Stem Cells," March/April 2008, p. 26

Funding for Alzheimer's Versus Other Diseases

Researchers have made amazing progress over the years in learning about Alzheimer's, and they are aggressively searching for its cause, ways to diagnose it in its earliest stages, improved treatments, and potentially a cure. Many of them are frustrated, however, because even though Alzheimer's cases are increasing exponentially, federal funding for Alzheimer's research is small compared with funding for many other diseases and disorders.

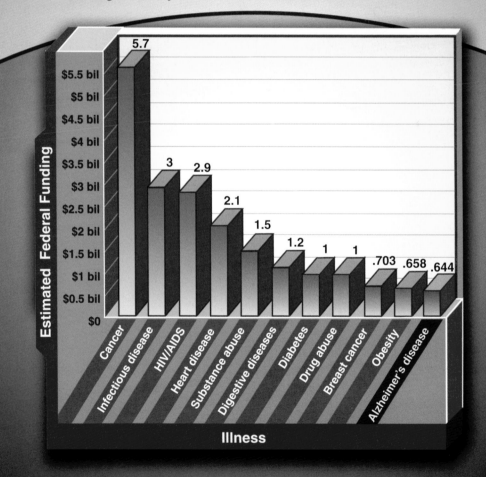

Source: National Institutes of Health, "Estimates of Funding for Various Diseases, Conditions, Research Areas," February 5, 2008. www.nih.gov.

States with Highest Increase in Alzheimer's Cases

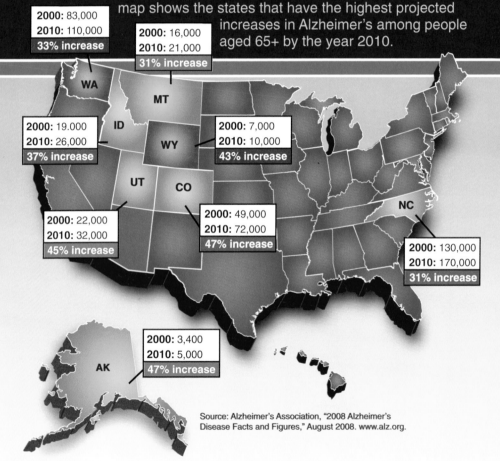

The number of people with Alzheimer's varies widely by state, as do projections for future growth in prevalence. According to the Alzheimer's Association, the reason some states will have higher increases than others is because of anticipated growth in their older populations, along with reduced mortality from other causes. This map shows the states that have the highest projected increases in Alzheimer's among people aged 65+ by the year 2010.

WA
2000: 83,000
2010: 110,000
33% increase

MT
2000: 16,000
2010: 21,000
31% increase

ID
2000: 19.000
2010: 26,000
37% increase

WY
2000: 7,000
2010: 10,000
43% increase

UT
2000: 22,000
2010: 32,000
45% increase

CO
2000: 49,000
2010: 72,000
47% increase

NC
2000: 130,000
2010: 170,000
31% increase

AK
2000: 3,400
2010: 5,000
47% increase

Source: Alzheimer's Association, "2008 Alzheimer's Disease Facts and Figures," August 2008. www.alz.org.

- In February 2008 researchers announced that a drug originally intended to counter arthritis symptoms was injected into an elderly physician suffering from Alzheimer's; afterward, the man showed **clearer thinking and was able to walk better.**

Sobering Predictions for the Future

Researchers have projected the number of new Alzheimer's cases that could occur in the future if current population trends remain steady. By the year 2050, if no preventive treatments or cures are found, there will be nearly 1 million new cases of Alzheimer's disease. Two factors will contribute to this large increase: the growing number of elderly people (especially those over 85), and the fact that risk of Alzheimer's increases as people get older. The annual number of new cases is expected to climb sharply around the year 2040 when all the baby boomers will be over the age of 65.

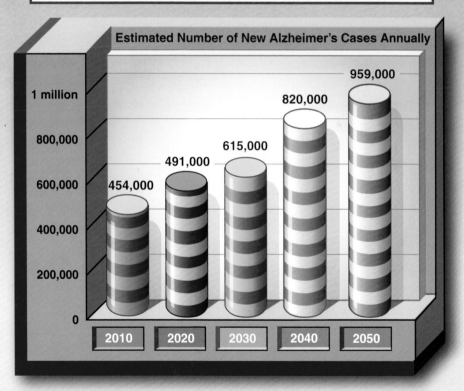

Estimated Number of New Alzheimer's Cases Annually

Source: National Institute on Aging, National Institutes of Health, "Alzheimer's Disease: Unraveling the Mystery," 2003.

- In April 2008 researchers at the University of Pittsburgh Medical Center announced the development of an imaging agent that attaches to brain areas damaged by Alzheimer's disease that may allow doctors to **diagnose Alzheimer's at an earlier stage**.

- German researchers announced in April 2008 that they had developed a potential cure for Alzheimer's, a technique that inhibits an enzyme known to be a main cause of brain decay; when used on mice, the creatures **did not succumb to the equivalent of Alzheimer's disease**.

- A study released in April 2008 by researchers at the University of California, Irvine, showed that an experimental Alzheimer's vaccine was effective in **clearing amyloid plaques** from the brains of aging dogs, but it **did not restore cognitive damage**.

- A study released in May 2008 showed that people who took the painkiller ibuprofen for more than 5 years had a **40 percent** lower risk of developing Alzheimer's disease.

- In October 2006 researchers from the Scripps Research Institute in La Jolla, California, reported that **THC**, the active ingredient in marijuana that produces the "high," may help **prevent the onset of Alzheimer's disease**.

Key People and Advocacy Groups

Alois Alzheimer: The German physician who discovered Alzheimer's disease and for whom it is named.

Alzheimer's Association: A leading voluntary health organization that seeks to eliminate Alzheimer's disease through research as well as to provide and enhance care and support for those who have the disease.

Michael J. Fox: A well-known television and film actor who suffers from Parkinson's disease and is a spokesperson on behalf of stem cell research as a possible cure for degenerative brain diseases.

Charlton Heston: A former president of the National Rifle Association and a well-known actor who suffered from Alzheimer's disease and died in 2008.

National Institute on Aging (NIA): The NIA supports and conducts research on aging processes, age-related diseases, and special problems and needs of the aged.

Terry Pratchett: A best-selling author of fantasy novels who was diagnosed with a rare form of early-onset Alzheimer's in December 2007; in May 2008 Pratchett announced that the disease was beginning to interfere with his writing.

Ronald Reagan: The fortieth president of the United States, who was diagnosed with Alzheimer's disease in 1994 and died in 2004.

Chronology

1907
German physician Alois Alzheimer publishes a paper about a "peculiar disease" that destroyed the brain of his patient, Auguste Deter.

1912
Solomon Carter Fuller, recognized as America's first black psychiatrist, publishes a comprehensive clinical review of all Alzheimer's cases that have been reported. He becomes the first to translate into English much of Alois Alzheimer's work on the disease.

1987
Actress Rita Hayworth, who is known for her battle with Alzheimer's, dies from Alzheimer's-related complications at the age of 68. Ronald Reagan praises her work in bringing Alzheimer's disease into the spotlight.

1980
The Alzheimer's Disease and Related Disorders Association is incorporated; later its name is changed to the Alzheimer's Association.

| 1900 | 1970 | 1980 | 1990 |

1910
Emil Kraepelin, known as "the Father of Modern Psychiatry," names the newly discovered disease after Alois Alzheimer.

1982
President Ronald Reagan designates the first National Alzheimer's Disease Awareness Week.

1992
Researchers identify a gene that is associated with the familial form of neurodegenerative disease.

Scientists from the National Institute of Neurological Disorders and Stroke isolate segments of DNA sequence that uniquely identify more than 2,300 brain genes.

1974
Congress grants authority to form the National Institute on Aging as a part of the National Institutes of Health. The new agency is charged with providing leadership in research and training, disseminating health information, and developing other programs that are relevant to aging and older people.

1993

The U.S. Food and Drug Administration approves the first drug for Alzheimer's, known as tacrine, which conserves the brain's supply of acetylcholine by slowing its breakdown.

2007

Best-selling British author Terry Pratchett announces that he has been diagnosed with early-onset Alzheimer's disease and donates $1 million to fund Alzheimer's research.

2002

The Alzheimer's Association estimates that 4 million people in the United States suffer from Alzheimer's disease.

President George W. Bush proclaims November to be National Alzheimer's Disease Awareness Month.

1995

2000

2005

1994

Ronald Reagan publicly announces that he has been diagnosed with Alzheimer's disease.

2004

At the age of 93, Ronald Reagan dies of Alzheimer's-related complications, which again puts the disease in the national spotlight and begins to create awareness of its severity.

2006

Researchers from Belgium are the first to show that the quantity of amyloid protein in brain cells is a major risk factor for Alzheimer's disease.

2008

Actor Charlton Heston dies from complications of Alzheimer's disease.

The Alzheimer's Association announces that the number of Americans with Alzheimer's disease has risen to 5.2 million and warns that prevalence could reach 16 million by 2050.

Related Organizations

Alzheimer's Association

225 N. Michigan Ave., 17th Floor

Chicago, IL 60601-7633

phone: (312) 335-8700 • toll-free fax: (866) 699-1246

e-mail: info@alz.org • Web site: www.alz.org

The Alzheimer's Association is a leading voluntary health organization that seeks to eliminate Alzheimer's disease through research as well as to provide and enhance care and support for those who have the disease. Numerous materials are available on its Web site, including news releases, journals such as *Alzheimer's & Dementia*, and a special section for kids and teens that has an interactive "brain tour."

Alzheimer's Disease Education and Referral (ADEAR) Center

PO Box 8250

Silver Spring, MD 20907-8250

phone: (301) 495-3311 • toll-free: (800) 438-4380

fax: (301) 495-3334

e-mail: adear@nia.nih.gov • Web site: www.alzheimers.nia.nih.gov

ADEAR, which is a service of the National Institute on Aging, serves health professionals, people with Alzheimer's disease and their families, and the general public by compiling, archiving, and distributing Alzheimer's-related information. Its Web site offers a number of informative materials, including the *Connections* newsletter and educational booklets called *Unraveling the Mystery* and *What Happens Next?*

Alzheimer's Foundation of America (AFA)

322 Eighth Ave., 7th Floor

New York, NY 10001

toll-free phone: (866) 232-8484 • fax: (646) 638-1546

e-mail: info@ alzfdn.org • Web site: www.alzfdn.org

The AFA's mission is "to provide optimal care and services" to those who are facing Alzheimer's or other types of dementia as well as to their caregivers and families through its member organizations that are dedicated to improving quality of life. Its Web site offers current and archived issues of the *Care ADvantage* magazine and *AFA Voices* newsletter as well as a wide variety of information about Alzheimer's disease.

American Health Assistance Foundation (AHAF)

22512 Gateway Center Dr.

Clarksburg, MD 20871

phone: (301) 948-3244 • toll-free: (800) 437-2423

fax: 301-258-9454

e-mail: info@ahaf.org • Web site: www.ahaf.org

The AHAF is a leading supporter of scientific and medical investigations into diseases that primarily affect the elderly, including Alzheimer's. Since the organization was founded in 1973, it has awarded more than $82 million in research grants to scientists working at universities, hospitals, and medical centers throughout the world. Publications available on its Web site include the *Alzheimer's Research Review* newsletter and the *Understanding Alzheimer's Disease* booklet as well as research information, videos, and medical illustrations.

Centers for Disease Control and Prevention (CDC)

1600 Clifton Rd.

Atlanta, GA 30333

phone: (404) 498-1515 • toll-free: (800) 311-3435

toll-free fax: (800) 553-6323

e-mail: inquiry@cdc.gov • Web site: www.cdc.gov

The CDC, which is part of the U.S. Department of Health and Human Services, is charged with promoting health and quality of life by controlling disease, injury, and disability. Its Web site offers a variety of Alzheimer's fact sheets, research papers, and information about the "Healthy Brain Initiative."

Family Caregiver Alliance/ National Center on Caregiving (FCA)

180 Montgomery St., Suite 1100

San Francisco, CA 94104

phone: (415) 434-3388 • toll-free: (800) 445-8106

fax: (415) 434-3508

e-mail: info@caregiver.org • Web site: www.caregiver.org

The FCA, an organization that seeks to address the needs of families and friends who provide long-term care at home, offers programs at national, state, and local levels to support caregivers. Available on its Web site are news releases, policy statements, fact sheets, research documents, and seven different e-newsletters.

Fisher Center for Alzheimer's Research Foundation

One Intrepid Sq.

W. 46th St. and 12th Ave.

New York, NY 10036

phone: (212) 957-7020 • toll-free: (800) 259-4636

fax: (212) 265-1075

e-mail: info@alzinfo.org • Web site: www.alzinfo.org

The Fisher Center for Alzheimer's Research Foundation, which funds more than 85 scientists throughout the United States, is dedicated to "attacking the scourge of Alzheimer's" by its focus on finding a cure and its support of educational programs. Its Web site offers numerous research publications as well as Alzheimer's disease news, information on causes and risk factors, diagnosis, and treatment.

John Douglas French Alzheimer's Foundation

11620 Wilshire Blvd., Suite 270

Los Angeles, CA 90025

phone: (310) 445-4650 • toll-free: (800) 477-2243

fax: (310) 479-0516

e-mail: jdfaf@earthlink.net • Web site: www.jdfaf.org

This organization's objective is to support cutting-edge research that can expedite the day when a cure for Alzheimer's disease is found. To accomplish that, it provides seed money for researchers and scientists in California who might not otherwise be funded. Its Web site offers a newsletter published each fall and spring as well as a number of research summaries.

National Institute of Mental Health (NIMH)

Science Writing, Press, and Dissemination Branch

6001 Executive Blvd., Room 8184, MSC 9663

Bethesda, MD 20892-9663

toll-free phone: (866) 615-6464 • fax: (301) 443-4279

e-mail: nimhinfo@nih.gov • Web site: www.nimh.nih.gov

The NIMH seeks to reduce mental illness and behavioral disorders through research and supports science that will profoundly affect the diagnosis, treatment, and prevention of mental disorders. The Web site's search engine links to numerous publications about Alzheimer's disease.

National Institute of Neurological Disorders and Stroke (NINDS)

PO Box 5801

Bethesda, MD 20824

phone: (301) 496-5751 • toll-free: (800) 352-9424

fax: (301) 402-2060

Web site: www.ninds.nih.gov

The NINDS, which is part of the National Institutes of Health, seeks to reduce the burden of neurological disease throughout the world through research and education. A number of publications are available on its Web site, including news articles, research papers, and general information about Alzheimer's disease.

National Institutes of Health (NIH)

9000 Rockville Pike

Bethesda, MD 20892

phone: (301) 496-4000

e-mail: nihinfo@od.nih.gov • Web site: www.nih.gov

The NIH, the leading medical research organization in the United States, is the primary federal agency for conducting and supporting medical research. NIH scientists search for ways to improve human health as well as investigate the causes, treatments, and possible cures for diseases. The Web site's MedLine Plus section offers a wide variety of links to Alzheimer's-related information.

National Organization for Rare Disorders (NORD)

55 Kenosia Ave.

PO Box 1968

Danbury, CT 06813-1968

phone: (203) 744-0100 • toll-free: (800) 999-6673 (voice mail only)

fax: (203) 798-2291

e-mail: orphan@rarediseases.org • Web site: www.rarediseases.org

NORD is committed to the identification, treatment, and cure of rare disorders (known as "orphan" diseases) through programs of education, advocacy, research, and service. Its Web site features a database of rare diseases, news articles, speeches and testimonies, and position papers.

For Further Research

Books

Marc E. Agronin, *Alzheimer's Disease and Other Dementias*. Philadelphia: Lippincott, Williams & Wilkins, 2008.

Rita Bresnahan, *Walking One Another Home: Moments of Grace and Possibility in the Midst of Alzheimer's*. Liguori, MO: Liguori/Triumph, 2003.

Eleanor Cooney, *Death in Slow Motion: A Memoir of a Mother, Her Daughter, and the Beast Called Alzheimer's*. New York: HarperCollins, 2003.

Paul Dash and Nicole Villemarette-Pittman, *Alzheimer's Disease*. New York: Demos Medical, 2005.

Ann Davidson, *A Curious Kind of Widow*. McKinleyville, CA: Fithian, 2006.

Thomas DeBaggio, *Losing My Mind: An Intimate Look at Life with Alzheimer's*. New York: Free Press, 2002.

Gayatri Devi and Deborah Mitchell, *What Your Doctor May Not Tell You About Alzheimer's Disease*. New York: Warner, 2004.

Healing Project, ed., *Voices of Alzheimer's*. Cambridge, MA: DaCapo Lifelong, 2004.

Lauren Kessler, *Finding Life in the Land of Alzheimer's*. New York: Penguin, 2008.

Pat Moffett, *Ice Cream in the Cupboard: A True Story of Early Onset Alzheimer's*. Garden City, NY: Morgan James, 2008.

Ronald Peterson, ed. *Mayo Clinic Guide to Alzheimer's Disease*. Rochester, MN: Mayo Clinic, 2006.

David Shenk, *The Forgetting: Alzheimer's; Portrait of an Epidemic*. New York: Anchor, 2003.

Richard Taylor, *Alzheimer's from the Inside Out*. Baltimore: Health Professions, 2007.

Periodicals

Sarah Baldauf, "A Father, a Dream, and Alzheimer's," *U.S. News & World Report*, May 26, 2008.

Michael Barbella, "Father's Death Inspires Pharmacist to Educate Others About Alzheimer's," *Drug Topics*, November 5, 2007.

Allison Flood, "'Humor Can Exist in the Most Dreadful Trials,'" *Bookseller*, April 18, 2008.

Christine Gorman, "Can You Prevent Alzheimer's Disease?" *Time*, January 16, 2006.

Christine Gorman et al., "The Fires Within," *Time*, February 23, 2004.

Denise Grady, "Finding Alzheimer's Before a Mind Fails," *New York Times*, December 26, 2007.

Jane Gross, "Living with Alzheimer's Before a Window Closes," *New York Times*, March 29, 2007.

Diane Guernsey, "What You Need to Know About Alzheimer's," *Town & Country*, November 2007.

Laurie Herr, "Jay's Story," *ELDR*, Spring 2008.

Robert Langreth, "Attacking Alzheimer's," *Forbes*, April 21, 2008.

Christine Larson, "Attacking Alzheimer's," *U.S. News & World Report*, February 11, 2008.

Jane L. Levere, "Opening Eyes to a Slowly Dimming World," *New York Times*, April 17, 2007.

Sandra Levy, "A Pharmacist and Dog in Tow Are Alzheimer's Patients' Best Friends," *Drug Topics*, November 19, 2007.

Steve Maich, "The Concussion Time Bomb," *Maclean's*, October 22, 2007.

January W. Payne, "Belly Fat Is Linked to Dementia Risk," *U.S. News & World Report*, March 26, 2008.

Andrew Pollack, "Scientists Report Advances in Diagnosing Alzheimer's Years Before Onset," *New York Times*, October 15, 2007.

Roni Caryn Rabin, "For a Sharp Brain, Stimulation," *New York Times*, May 13, 2008.

Claude Solnik, "Alzheimer's Invisible Victims," *Long Island (NY) Business News*, May 2, 2008.

Dianne Tow, "Music Is Magic for Residents with Alzheimer's," *Nursing Homes*, November 2006.

Internet Sources

Manny Alvarez, "Alzheimer's Disease: Betrayed by Your Brain," Fox News, February 21, 2007. www.foxnews.com/story/0,2933,253541,00.html?sPage=fnc/health/longevity.

Alzheimer's Association, "2008 Alzheimer's Disease Facts and Figures," August2008.www.alz.org/national/documents/report_alzfactsfigures 2008.pdf.

Patti Davis, "Letting Go," *Newsweek*, November 14, 2007. www.news week.com/id/70463.

Craig Freudenrich, "How Your Brain Works," How Stuff Works. www.howstuffworks.com/brain.htm.

Barbara Kantrowitz and Karen Springen, "Confronting Alzheimer's," *Newsweek*, August 21, 2007. www.newsweek.com/id/34002.

National Institute on Aging, *Alzheimer's Disease: Unraveling the Mystery*, December 2003. www.nia.nih.gov/NR/rdonlyres/A294D332-71A 2-4866-BDD7-A0DF216DAAA4/0/Alzheimers_Disease_Unravel ing_the_Mystery.pdf.

Lauran Neergaard, "O'Connor Makes Personal Plea for Alzheimer's Aid," *Washington Post*, May 14, 2008. www.washingtonpost.com/wp-dyn/content/article/2008/05/14/AR2008051400373.html?nav=hcmodule.

PBS *Online NewsHour*, "Stealing Minds," June 8, 2004. www.pbs.org/newshour/bb/remember/jan-june04/minds_06-08.html.

Terry Pratchett, "Boomers' Little Secret," *Newsweek International*, April 21, 2008. www.newsweek.com/id/131711.

Source Notes

Overview

1. Quoted in American Presidents: Life Portraits, "Letters: Ronald Reagan," November 5, 1994. www.americanpresidents.org.
2. Terry Pratchett, "An Embuggerance," *DiscWorld News*, December 11, 2007. www.paulkidby.com.
3. Rudolph Tanzi, "An Interview with Dr. Rudolph Tanzi," China Millennium Council, 2005. www.chinafrontier.com.
4. Alzheimer's Association, "2008 Alzheimer's Disease Facts and Figures," August 2008. www.alz.org.
5. Alzheimer's Association, "2008 Alzheimer's Disease Facts and Figures."
6. Ruth A. Brandwein, "Mom Had Alzheimer's," in *Voices of Alzheimer's,* ed. Healing Project. Cambridge, MA: DaCapo Lifelong, 2004, p. 73.
7. Richard Taylor, *Alzheimer's from the Inside Out*. Baltimore: Health Professions, 2007, p. 34.
8. National Institute on Aging, "The Changing Brain in Alzheimer's Disease," August 29, 2006. www.nia.nih.gov.
9. Quoted in Shankar Vedantam, "Mind Games May Trump Alzheimer's," *Washington Post*, June 19, 2003, p. A1.
10. Madison Institute of Health, "How Is Alzheimer's Disease Treated?" 2008. http://alzheimers.factsforhealth.org.
11. Quoted in Rebecca Rosenberg, "Experts Prescribe Children's Toys for Alzheimer's Patients," Columbia News Service, April 24, 2007. http://jscms.jrn.columbia.edu.
12. National Institute on Aging, "Finding New Answers and Asking Better Questions," *Unraveling the Mystery*, August 29, 2006. www.nia.nih.gov.

How Does Alzheimer's Disease Affect the Brain?

13. Quoted in Konrad Mauer, Stephan Volk, and Hector Gerbaldo, "Auguste D and Alzheimer's Disease," *Lancet*, May 24, 1997, p. 1,548.
14. National Institute on Aging, "Inside the Human Brain," November 26, 2007. www.nia.nih.gov.
15. Alzheimer's Association, "Basics of Alzheimer's Disease," 2005. www.alz.org.
16. Sam Gandy, "Families Advocate for Alzheimer's Disease to Be National Priority," PBS *Online NewsHour*, July 26, 2006. www.pbs.org.
17. Mayo Clinic, "Destroyed Nerve Cells: A Future for Lost Memory," 2008. http://discoverysedge.mayo.edu.
18. Merle Comer, "Families Advocate for Alzheimer's Disease to Be National Priority," PBS NewsHour, July 26, 2006. www.pbs.org.
19. Ron Wheeler, interview with author, May 27, 2008.
20. Wheeler, interview.
21. Wheeler, interview.
22. Wheeler, interview.

What Causes Alzheimer's Disease?

23. Quoted in Mike Falcon, "Anne Archer Aims for Alzheimer's Cure," *USA Today*, November 21, 2001. www.usatoday.com.
24. Ronald Peterson, ed., *Mayo Clinic on Alzheimer's Disease*. Rochester, MN: Mayo Clinic Health Information, 2002, p. 43.

25. National Institute on Aging, "Alzheimer's Disease Genetics," August 2004. www.nia.nih.gov.

26. Quoted in ABC News, "Link Between Heart Disease, Alzheimer's," January 14, 2008. http://abcnews.go.com.

27. Quoted in *Forbes*, "Heart Disease a Risk Factor for Alzheimer's," June 10, 2007. www.forbes.com.

28. Quoted in Stuart Jeffries, "'There's Humour in the Darkest Places,'" *Guardian*, March 18, 2008. http://books.guardian.co.uk.

Who Suffers from Alzheimer's Disease?

29. Thomas DeBaggio, *Losing My Mind: An Intimate Look at Life with Alzheimer's*. New York: Free Press, 2002, p. 3.

30. Quoted in Johns Hopkins Bloomberg School of Public Health, "Alzheimer's Disease to Quadruple Worldwide by 2050," news release, June 10, 2007. www.jhsph.edu.

31. Daniel Pendick, "The Color of Risk," *Memory Loss & the Brain*, Winter 2008. www.memorylossonline.com/winter 2008.

32. Alzheimer's Association, "2008 Alzheimer's Disease Facts and Figures."

33. Quoted in Curtis Krueger, "Alzheimer's, Down's Link Sheds Light," *St. Petersburg (FL) Times*, March 10, 2008. www.sptimes.com.

34. Quoted in Krueger, "Alzheimer's, Down's Link Sheds Light."

35. Colin Davidson, "Ask a Geneticist," *Understanding Genetics*, July 13, 2004. www.thetech.org.

36. Quoted in Jenna Sloan and Lucy Laing, "Tragic Six-Year-Old Is Struck Down with Alzheimer's Disease," *Daily Mirror* (London), January 31, 2008. www.mirror.co.uk.

37. Quoted in Kate Devlin, "Boy, 2, Suffers from Children's Alzheimer's," *Daily Telegraph* (London), May 8, 2008. www.telegraph.co.uk.

38. Patti Davis, "Letting Go," *Newsweek*, November 14, 2007. www.newsweek.com.

39. Brenda van Dyck, "Losing My Father," in *Voices of Alzheimer's*, pp. 91, 93.

Will Research Prevent or Cure Alzheimer's Disease?

40. Maria Torroella Carney, "Alzheimer's Disease and a Look to the Future," in *Voices of Alzheimer's*, p. 249.

41. Quoted in Sam Jaffe, "An Eye Test for Alzheimer's," *Wired*, February 6, 2002. www.wired.com.

42. Quoted in *Science Daily*, "Detecting Alzheimer's Early," December 1, 2005. www.sciencedaily.com.

43. Edward L. Tobinick and Hyman Gross, "Rapid Cognitive Improvement in Alzheimer's Disease Following Perispinal Etanercept Administration," *Journal of Neuroinflammation*, January 2008. www.nrimed.com.

44. Larry Goldstein, "Testimony of Larry Goldstein, Ph.D, Regarding 'Exploring the Promise of Embryonic Stem Cell Research,'" June 8, 2005. www.isscr.org.

45. Quoted in William J. Cromie, "Stem Cells Reduce Brain Damage," *Harvard University Gazette*, November 21, 2002. www.hno.harvard.edu.

46. John C. Morris, "Readers' Questions: Alzheimer's Disease," *New York Times*, December 26, 2007. http://science.blogs.nytimes.com.

List of Illustrations

Index

acetylcholine, 18

African Americans, prevalence of Alzheimer's among, 54–55

age, as greatest risk factor for developing Alzheimer's, 38, 48, 50 (chart)

aluminum, development of Alzheimer's and, 42

Alvarez, Manny, 45

Alzheimer, Alois, 20–21

Alzheimer Society of Canada, 46

Alzheimer's Association, 20, 64, 77
  on operation of neurons, 20
  on prevalence of Alzheimer's disease, 53, 60
  on projected increase in Alzheimer's cases, 7, 13
  on risk of developing Alzheimer's, 38

Alzheimer's disease
  affects on brain, 10–12, 32, 34 (illustration), 35 (illustration)
  association with Down syndrome, 55–57, 65
  chronic diseases and risk for, 40–41
  costs of, 81
  diagnosis of, 16, 44, 85
    advances in, 70–71
    using MRI, 81
  early-onset, 9–10, 39, 47
    vs. late onset type, 9–10
  environmental factors and, 41–43
  factors in development of, 49 (illustration)
  fear of, 67 (chart)
  medical conditions associated with, 51 (chart)
  prevalence of, 6, 12–13, 53–54, 60, 61
    aging population and, 59, 62
  projection of annual new cases of, 85 (chart)
  risk factors for, 48

risk for, among minorities, 54–55

role of genetics in, 38–40

stages of, 13–14, 16

symptoms of, 7

treatment of, 7, 17–19

Alzheimer's Research Foundation, 61

American Health Assistance Foundation, 29, 30

Ames, David, 62

amyloid precursor protein, 23

Archives of Neurology (journal), 55

Barnes, Carol, 62

beta-amyloid plaques, 6, 24, 32
  detection of, in eye, 70

brain
  affects of Alzheimer's disease on, 10–12
  Alzheimer's, changes in, 34 (illustration), 35 (illustration)
  shrinkage in, 32
  structure and function of, 21–22, 33 (illustration)

brain stem, 22

Brandwein, Ruth A., 13–14

Brookmeyer, Ron, 54

Carney, Maria Torroella, 69–70

Centers for Disease Control and Prevention (CDC), 9, 68

cerebellum, 22

cerebral cortex, 22

cerebrum, 21–22

cholesterol
  apolipoprotein E gene and, 39
  caffeine and, 50
  high levels of, as risk for Alzheimer's, 12, 41, 54

cholinesterase inhibitors, 18

Cognitive Neurology and Alzheimer's Disease Center, 46

About the Author

Peggy J. Parks holds a bachelor of science degree from Aquinas College in Grand Rapids, Michigan, where she graduated magna cum laude. She is an author who has written more than 70 nonfiction educational books for children and young adults and has self-published her own cookbook, *Welcome Home: Recipes, Memories, and Traditions from the Heart*. Parks lives in Muskegon, Michigan, a town that she says inspires her writing because of its location on the shores of Lake Michigan.